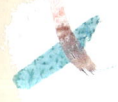

NEUROSIS IN SOCIETY

NEUROSIS IN SOCIETY

ANDREW SIMS
Professor of Psychiatry
University of Leeds

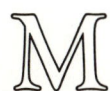

First published 1983 by
THE MACMILLAN PRESS LTD
London and Basingstoke
Companies and representatives throughout the world

Printed in Hong Kong

ISBN 0 333 33514 7 (hard cover)
      0 333 33515 5 (paper cover)

Contents

Foreword

by
The Lord Taylor of Harlow, MD, FRCP, FRCGP, FFL

Good clinical medicine, whether it is concerned with body or mind, starts with the careful observation of disease patterns. Only when the natural history of a disease episode has been established can prognosis be reliable and the effect of treatment properly assessed.

Professor Andrew Sims is a naturalist-psychiatrist in the tradition of Thomas Sydenham. For many years, he has been observing the nature, varieties and course of psychiatric illness, with a special interest in the severe neuroses. He has established beyond doubt that the severe neuroses are serious and intractable diseases, which carry with them a substantial mortality risk, even if suicide is excluded. He has observed and charted the close interaction between neurosis and the community whether it be the wider community of work and society, or the closer community of the family. Within these frames of reference, he has reviewed the full range of possible treatment, to see how far each technique yields results which are acceptable both socially and medically.

In this important book, he records his own observations, set against the published experience of many others. Severe neurosis is a subject of great difficulty. Any clear account is bound to be controversial if only because of the volume and diversity of speculative thinking in this field. Professor Sims sweeps through this confusion without being caught up in any particular dogma. He checks each assertion against the natural history of neurosis as he knows it, but leaves the reader to draw his own conclusions.

I have enjoyed particularly his accounts of the social neuroses, for example those caused by, or associated with, the Birmingham IRA bomb episodes. Today, he sees the epidemic neuroses spreading more rapidly than ever before, with the mass media as the vectors. He points out the mixed nature of many neuroses, with obsessional or hysterical features mixed with anxiety and depression. He quite rightly sees reactive or exogenous depression as a neurotic illness, the treatment of which is extremely difficult.

This is a book of great significance, to be read and pondered over by psychiatrists, physicians and general practitioners, as well as by those of the professions supplementary to medicine who have to deal with the neurotic in society. It should do much to improve the quality of care and understanding which the neurotic in society receives. It should also provide a springboard for further research, in particular for epidemiological studies. Sound epidemiology is the great enemy of unsound clinical speculation. The clear and honest picture which Professor Sims has painted provides a sound foundation on which future investigation of this difficult subject can be built.

House of Lords and Glyn Ceiriog, North Wales, 1982

1 What is Neurosis?

'Wer ther a Physitian that could cure the maladies of the mind,
as well as those of the body, he needed not to wish the Lord
Maior, or the Pope for his Uncle, for he should have patients
without number.'

James Howell, 1645, Epistolae
Ho-Elianae. Familia letters
domestic and forren

(See figure 1.1)

This is a book about that unfortunate person, the neurotic; not
about him (or her) in isolation but about how he gets on with his
family and friends, and the people he rubs shoulders with in the street
— 'society'. It is descriptive, a travel book if you like, but a journey
you have made as well as I. Perhaps yours was only the occasional
fleeting visit; your neurotic patient who was in hospital for manage-

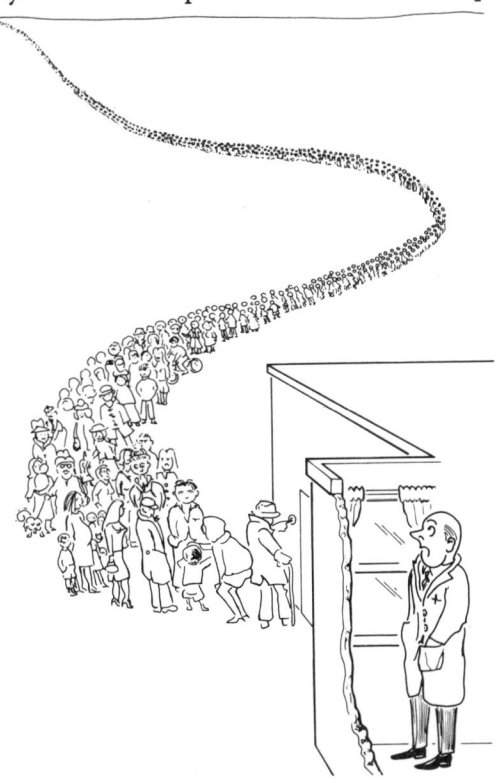

Figure 1.1   'Patients without number'

ment of his congestive cardiac failure; your divorced client who could not manage on supplementary benefit, and so took it out on you, her social worker. Such uncomfortable acquaintance with neurosis is shown in this letter from a general practitioner to a consultant psychiatrist.

>   The Surgery,
>   Market Street,
>   Bradfield.

Dr. B. Worryless,

Consultant Psychiatrist,

St. Belinda's Hospital.

Dear Dr. Worryless,

<u>re Miss Delia Panick, aged 31</u>

I would be grateful for your opinion of this young woman. She complains of dizziness and headaches and feels tired and limp. She lives with her mother and they quarrel all the time. Mother is a determined, bossy woman. She gets very irritated with Delia whom she criticizes and belittles for being useless.

Delia stopped going to work as a typist in the office of a big department store when her boss moved her to the middle of the room from her previous place beside the wall. She objects because she feels that she is going to fall off her chair! She has never done so, but she feels shaky and panics.

Her father died when she was 17 and she was very upset for a long time then, being off work for 2 years. She has had no steady boyfriend but used to go to a Singles Group. She has stopped going because she feels frightened to leave the house. She has had dates via a Marriage Bureau but says, "most of them take one look at me and say 'no'".

I don't know what can be done to help her - if anything.

>   Yours sincerely,
>   John Healthwright.

We will look first at neurosis in different populations; neurosis is important to those concerned to help, because it is so common. We will then use a higher power of the microscope and examine it clinically, looking at the phenomena of neuroses and personality disorders. What does the person actually experience? How does he view his difficulties? Finally treatment is discussed in general principle, without going into the intricacies of psychotherapy or behaviour therapy. The aim is to show how treatment can be applied to prevent the natural history of neurosis becoming inevitable; to see how intervention can prevent deterioration and help motivate the individual sufferer towards improvement.

Definition and Meaning

Neurosis is a psychological reaction to acute or continuous perceived stress, expressed in emotion or behaviour ultimately inappropriate in dealing with that stress.

Illness or Reaction

In several respects neurosis is unique amongst 'diseases'. Is it a disease at all? It has no organic basis and the patient often has insight into his problems. The most common of the mental conditions, one of the most common afflictions of mankind and treated by the general practitioner, it has no constant form, so that it is often defined by exclusion. It is a state of sustained mental and emotional discomfort of such abnormal intensity as to interfere with an individual's adjustment to everyday life.

Is it 'illness' or 'a reaction'? At first sight this question seems to be of fundamental importance. If it is an illness it should have a described pathology, be referred to doctors and treated medically. If it is not an illness but a psychological or social reaction it should not be referred to doctors but should be dealt with by psychologists, social workers, community workers, personnel officers or priests. In practice it is dealt with by doctors, and by all these other professional workers as well, and there still remain plenty more sufferers from neurosis who have not made contact with any of the cohort of helpers.

A 35-year-old woman with a responsible job in broadcasting complained bitterly of pain in her jaw that had lasted 15 years. She had received many different surgical and dental treatments. She was incapacitated in that she had difficulty in talking clearly and could only eat sloppy foods. Although her upbringing had been very disturbed, no definite conflict was demonstrated to which this could be a psychological reaction. Although no organic explanation could be found, her pain and loss of function justified the term 'illness'.

Boundaries of Neurosis

If I have painted a picture of a very vague, ill-defined condition that would be a mistake. It is ill-defined but not vague; that is to say, it is often difficult to determine what is neurosis and what is something else. But at its core neurosis is a meaningful term which merits description. A geographical analogy could be drawn with the state and nation of Poland. If the State of Poland is compared in 1880, 1930 and 1980, the frontiers are seen to have expanded enormously in 1930 compared with 50 years before, and then by the third date the whole country has moved a hundred or so miles to the West. Because of its fluctuating boundaries this does not make Poland, or to be Polish, a vague idea; any Pole would make eloquent denial of that.

A comparable 'geographical' model for neurosis is shown in figure 1.2. The borders between neurosis and other conditions are blurred at certain points. The widest and most indefinite interfaces occur: (1) in that broad hinterland either side of a purely arbitrary frontier between neurosis and personality disorder; (2) where the 'subclinical neurotic syndrome' marches with normality (Who is not neurotic?); (3) where mood disturbance is neither clearly neurotic nor exclusively

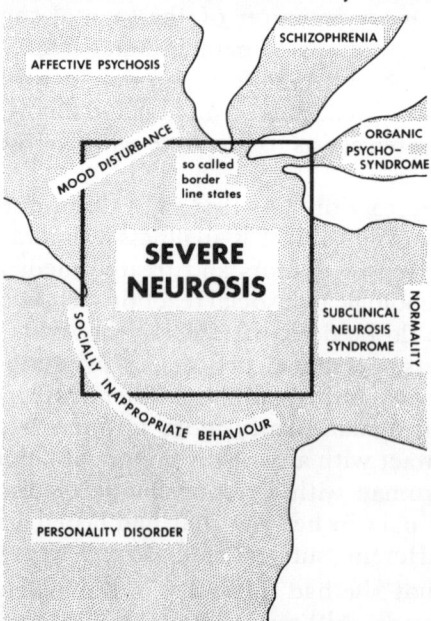

Figure 1.2   Geographical model of neurosis

relevant to 'affective psychosis'. In practice, of course, an operational definition will create arbitrary boundaries for the concept, rather like the frontiers of a state: they are practically important although non-sensical in terms of physical geography. So, in figure 1.2, the operational definition for my concept of *severe neurosis* will be a sharply defined box rather to the 'west' of subclinical neurosis, and will include those patients requiring treatment in hospital for neurosis without any other non-neurotic diagnosis. A general practitioner investigating neurosis in his practice population would probably include a population shifted to the 'east' and including much of the subclinical neurosis syndrome. A psychologist employed by the Home Office to evaluate a prison population might be concentrating on a more 'southerly' group with an emphasis on personality disorder, where the behaviour of subjects impairs their relationships with individuals and society.

In this figure the differentiation of neurosis from schizophrenia, or neurosis from organic states is generally simple. There are a few situations, such as where head injury is complicated by an hysterical reaction, in which it is difficult to decide whether neurosis is present or not, but this is a rarer problem than the differential diagnosis from normality, personality disorder or depression. The distinction from schizophrenia has not usually proved a common problem in British psychiatry; in North America, where the term *schizophrenia* is used more widely, differentiation is sometimes difficult and *borderline state* or *schizophrenia spectrum disorder* is described. Sometimes, of course, neurosis and schizophrenia, or neurosis and an organic state coincide; to return to our analogy above, a person, because of his parentage and place of birth, may be both a Pole and a Slovak. As this book proceeds it will become apparent that there is no absolute and logical separation between neurosis and personality disorder.

The Characteristics of Normality

All of us are neurotic; most of us know ourselves to be neurotic inside ourselves; some are more neurotic than others. The following are descriptions of neurotic patterns of thought, but a normal person may occasionally feel these emotions also: (1) a lack of self-acceptance and low self-esteem in which he sees himself as ineffectual, deficient, immature or even deformed as a person; (2) a dichotomy between 'myself as I know myself to be' and the fantasy self 'I wish I were'; (3) a desperate attempt to hold himself together against overpowering forces of disintegration in a hostile world and a meaningless universe; (4) a longing to belong with, at the same time, a self-centred, self-conscious barrier preventing him freely relating to others; (5) a lack of ability to give or receive love in the amount he would like despite his aspirations otherwise.

What is the difference between normal and neurotic? It is partly in degree, and partly in the behaviour that results from this internal clamour. The neurotic claims to feel this state of dis-ease all the time or most of the time. He does not find this discomfort a stimulus to work for something better, but rather it is a dense fog that completely prevents his seeing any solution that he could use. He searches but with little hope of enlightenment.

A middle-aged schoolmaster consults his general practitioner complaining of muscular pains in his left shoulder, irritability and difficulty in getting off to sleep. The doctor reassures him and prescribes a mild sedative for three weeks until the next school holiday; the symptoms clear without further intervention. Out of interest the doctor consults his records and finds that this man has consulted seven times in the last two years, always during term time and always a fresh somatic complaint. It is an almost arbitrary decision whether the doctor considers this to be a *neurotic* reaction in a basically *normal* person, or a neurotic illness.

Neurosis is different from an illness like pneumonia or schizophrenia that one either has or has not. It is possible to have a 'touch' of neurosis, and there is no absolute demarcation between neurosis and normality. In this particular property it is similar to such conditions as hypertension, diabetes mellitus or epilepsy, all of which are considered to be present when some arbitrary limit has been passed. The greater the stress, the greater is the vulnerability to neurosis.

Psychosis and Neurosis

Although there is much argument, psychiatric classification still starts with the fundamental distinction between psychosis and neurosis. Psychoses are 'mental disorders in which impairment of mental function had developed to a degree that interferes grossly with insight, ability to meet some ordinary demands of life or to maintain adequate contact with reality' (World Health Organization, 1977).

Neurotic disorders 'are mental disorders without any demonstrable organic basis in which the patient may have considerable insight and has unimpaired reality testing, in that he usually does not confuse his morbid subjective experiences and fantasies with external reality. Behaviour may be greatly affected although usually remaining within socially acceptable limits, but personality is not disorganized' (World Health Organization, 1977).

These definitions describe fundamental differences between the two conditions for reality testing and insight, and also affect, behaviour, and social functioning. The psychotic is recognised as suffering from something quite outside our normal experience — it is ultimately not understandable. The neurotic is understood as being like us in our doubts and conflicts, only more so. Two patients both believed that their workmates were against them. One believed that the Freemasons were involved in a plot to poison him — the psychotic. The other, after complaining about his colleagues, in a moment of rare insight said, 'but then I should think I am pretty difficult to work alongside' — the neurotic.

Operational and Epidemiological Definition

To answer the question, 'What is neurosis?', one needs to investigate how neurosis occurs in populations. When neurosis is looked at with an epidemiological eye, the number of cases, their presentation and distribution is related to environmental conditions; that is neurosis is investigated in vivo rather than in vitro, in society rather than in the out-patient waiting room. Neurosis is chameleon-like and changes its colouring to take on characteristics imposed by society, and so its presentation in one environment will have different features from that in another. An operational definition is chosen to suit the particular group of people or 'population' that is being studied. In a study of a new town population, for example, incipient or *subclinical* *neurosis* was defined as the presence of four symptoms in a sample of people interviewed at home. The symptoms were *nerves*, depression, undue irritability and sleeplessness.

With different target populations, those attending their general practitioner, or those receiving treatment from hospital, different aspects of neurosis will be given a varying emphasis. However, the differences are usually of severity and distribution of symptoms; there are some symptoms common to all neuroses. Feelings of lack of energy and sleep difficulties are particularly prominent in the presentation of neurosis to the general practitioner, whilst housebound housewives, because of the nature of their complaint, are less likely to arrive at his consulting room.

The greatest severity of neurotic symptoms is found, appropriately enough, in those patients who are referred by their general practitioner to a psychiatrist. These probably only represent about 10% of the population at risk. There is a tendency for in-patients to be more severely neurotically disturbed than day patients, who are more disordered than those treated as out patients (Sims, 1976). About a third of the population appear to take more complaints to their general practitioner — these are described later under the *subclinical* *neurosis syndrome*. There are a few people (perhaps 16%) who do not describe emotional symptoms, even on specific enquiry. In figure 1.3 these different populations are represented graphically.

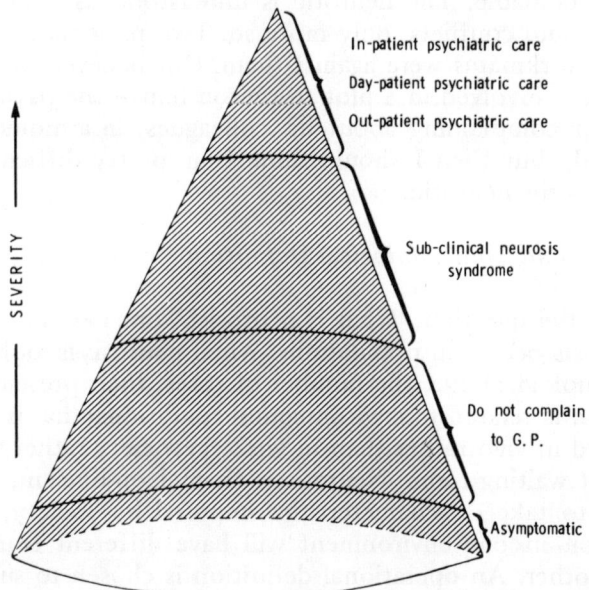

Figure 1.3   The neurotic cone: an epidemiological model. The approximate proportion of the population is represented by the volume of the cone

Behavioural and Symptomatic Definition

From a behavioural standpoint it is what he actually does (or perhaps does not), rather than the patient's internal mental state which receives prime attemtion. The emphasis is upon his deficiencies in social skills rather than on his feelings of isolation from other people.

Neurosis can be considered as maladaptive behaviour, a failure of coping mechanisms, an inappropriate method of dealing with externally or internally imposed stress. Behaviourists tend to concentrate on the fact that this particular item of behaviour, or this behaviour pattern, is maladaptive; that is, it does not achieve the goals which the person intends, or will benefit from. In contrast medicine, and hence psychiatry, has traditionally concentrated on symptoms for making a diagnosis, and so what the patient complains of, how he describes his difficulties with coping is regarded as important.

This emphasis on understanding symptoms and how it feels to be the sufferer 'inside himself' involves the skilled use of 'empathy'. The doctor tries to understand the sufferer's experience well enough to feel it so poignantly, that when he describes these symptoms back to the patient, the latter says, 'Yes, that is how I feel'.

Individual and Social Definition

Neurosis is a public and a private condition. It affects the person, how he feels inside himself, and it also influences his approach to other people and his relationship with them. It is an individual problem with social implications affecting the way he reacts to his immediate environment. His fear of losing his own identity makes him desperate to maintain it (unlike the psychotic who may lose his sense of identity with or without fear) and this reveals itself as a sort of selfishness, in which other people's needs are ignored.

As well as individual problems and symptoms affecting other people, it also works the other way. The tensions within society impinge upon and damage the individual. Neurosis distorts social relationships; it also arises as a result of society's unreasonable demands upon a person.

Neurosis is not a 'thing' in itself, but more one way of looking at thought or behaviour, in the same way that 'heads' or 'tails' are not 'things' as far as a coin is concerned, but simply aspects of the same whole, the way one person sees it from his side of the coin. So neurosis is the way professionals involved may conceptualise certain behaviour patterns, or particular self-descriptions of distress. There are advantages in describing this state of mankind in this particular way. First, it makes a distinction from other mental and physical problems that reach doctors, and second it emphasises the causal relationship with provoking stresses.

Why is Neurosis Important?

There are two factors that determine the importance of a disease; these are severity and commonness. Neurosis is extremely common. It is also important as an identifiable cause of human suffering. The neurotic describes himself as miserable, ineffective, lacking in achievement and gratification. He often feels incapable of action. We will discuss how neurosis is associated with physical illness and death. The neurotic is worse off than other people in a variety of different ways.

The neurotic's condition affects other people. A neurotic way of thinking, and neurotic interpretations of other people hinders easy relationships, damaging all areas of social life. There is impairment of effectiveness and relationships made at work. It also affects marriage, choice of spouse, the relationship the partners have within the marriage, the behaviour and demeanour of the neurotic's spouse and their sexual relationship. Neurosis has an intimate effect upon the family and the bringing up of children. It has repercussions in human history, in politics and in economic affairs. So the distorted way the person sees himself and his place in society involves his own immediate environment, and in proportion to his own influence it may have much wider implications. These social effects of neurosis have often been ignored and yet they are clearly important.

Once we have an idea of what neurosis is, the next stage is to describe its component parts, to understand what one is dealing with and to subdivide into rational categories. Even the most elementary taxonomy is still in doubt as neurotics may change from one sort of clinical picture to another in a fluid and unpredictable way. Today's anxiety state may change into tomorrow's phobic neurosis. The patient admitted to the day hospital because she is unable to leave the house may show no such symptoms in two weeks time but be describing major problems within her marriage. We still have the time-honoured but also time-expired traditional categories (anxiety state, hysteria, etc.). These represent a clinical description at a point in time but they are, to some extent, interchangeable and not mutually exclusive.

Prevalence in the Whole Community

Neurosis contributes a major part to many of the syndromes of folk lore without organic basis. One such condition was described to me by an old farmer in Mid-Wales as 'Clwy edau wlân', that is the 'disease of the woollen threads'. The patient suffers from lack of energy, listlessness, difficulty with sleep and generally feeling unwell. He would consult a local practitioner, of whom my informant knew two, both in their 70's, and the practitioner would measure the patient's wrist to elbow three times with a length of sheep's wool. If the length of wool was more than three cubits, then the diagnosis was confirmed, and the practitioner predicted that, without appropriate treatment, jaundice would occur. Treatment involved the village blacksmith acting as a medical ancillary, and he was paid 6d to drop a piece of newly forged steel into the patient's beer. Treatment was so effective that jaundice very rarely supervened. In time the patient usually lost his symptoms as well! The commonness of this condition, the fact that it produced a rather indefinite mixture of psychological and somatic symptoms without organic basis, the age and sex of the sufferers, and the natural history would suggest that this was in fact a form of neurosis. This account of symptoms can probably be matched, although in less dramatic form, in many other cultural groups.

Various quantitative estimates of neurosis have been made. One fairly constant finding is that women are more frequently affected than men, usually in a ratio of about 2:1. When this sex discrepancy is diminished, it is of interest to ascertain what are the local cultural conditions accounting for this. Here are the findings of some general population studies.

Stirling County Survey

How to distinguish pathological from a normal degree of neurosis is a difficult research problem. In community studies the proportion of the population labelled 'neurotic' is wholly determined by the operational definition for neurosis used. In the Stirling County Survey (Leighton *et al.*, 1963), in Maritime Canada, more than 1000 home interviews and other investigations found clear psychiatric disorder in 40% of women and 21% of men; only 17% of the population were free of disorder. This was a community survey and these people were not consulting a psychiatrist, yet more than half showed probable neurotic symptoms. Twenty per cent of this population were thought to be in need of psychiatric help and this corresponded very closely with a study in New York in which 23.4% of the Manhattan population in the Midtown study showed 'serious' symptoms (Srole, 1962).

In Stirling County it was found that with increasing age, with lower social class, and lower educational attainment, there was increasing likelihood of psychiatric disorder. Communities with low morale had higher rates for disorder and the usual excess of females compared with males affected tended to be reversed. From this study it can be seen that the more stringent the requiremtnts for a diagnosis of neurosis the fewer people will be placed within the category of 'disorder'.

Subclinical Neurosis Syndrome

We have already made brief allusion to another interesting study concerned with the frequency of neurosis in the general population. This was the classical investigation of health in Harlow New Town carried out by Taylor and Chave (1964). Harlow, in rural Essex, was built to relieve overcrowding in Central London, and a large number of young families were offered accommodation and employment in the town. Old people, single people and those who were chronically physically disabled or suffering from psychotic illness were markedly under-represented in the immigrants to Harlow. Most couples moving to the New Town had young children, and the birth rate in the first few years was very high. There were ample amenities provided in the town, but there was very little in common with the culture of the surrounding countryside.

Moving house for these people, most of whom had spent all their lives in the bustle of the big city, was understandably stressful. There was no longer the intimate network of social life in densely populated streets, with public houses at the street corners, and the habit of neighbourliness and close contact across the generations. They also lacked help from their own parents in bringing up young children.

The investigation of the population in Harlow New Town was carried out by trained interviewers visiting people at home in a random sample of households in the New Town. The population could be divided into two categories; those whose adaptation into their new community had been successful, and those who were presenting problems. These had more complaints about their social state at interview; they made more demands upon their general practitioners and upon hospital services; they also showed considerably more difficulty in adapting to the New Town conditions and required more help from the Housing Authorities and others concerned with the process of assimilation.

This third of the New Town population with more problems were designated *subclinical neurosis syndrome*. The proportion with subclinical neurosis syndrome was found to be similar in the Inner London Borough from which the New Town population had come, and also a London suburb. It would seem that those neurotically predisposed took their neurosis with them into changing circumstances. It had not been a bar to their moving, but it had caused them to have greater difficulties in adapting to new surroundings. In fact neurotics may show greater social mobility than the non-neurotic portion of the population because the neurotic's internal restlessness, which is partly caused by dissatisfaction with himself, may find expression in his running away from his present circumstances in search of a more congenial way of life.

Most of the new town population were in good health; the 'hard' indices including the adjusted death rate, and infant and maternal mortality rates, were all lower in the New Town than for England and Wales as a whole. Four symptoms of minor psychiatric ill health which showed a tendency to cluster were 'nerves', depression, undue irritability and sleeplessness, and these constituted *subclinical neurosis syndrome*. Length of residence in the New Town had no effect on the rate at which these nervous symptoms were reported in this third of the town's population. Symptoms and difficulties with adjustment are summarised in table 1.1.

More of the subclinical neurosis syndrome group spent more time at home, and more disliked staying at home than the rest of the New Town population.

*Table 1.1   Symptoms and social adjustment in new town residents with sub-
clinical neurosis syndrome (after Taylor and Chave)*

	Subclinical Neurosis Syndrome	Non-neurotic subjects
Mean consultations with general practitioner p.a.	5.2	3.5
Treated by G.P. for neurosis	12%	4%
Subjects considered that their health was good	55%	84%
Complained of loneliness	44%	17%
Boredom	53%	29%

Prevalence in Camberwell

Other studies have assessed the frequency of emotional disturbance
in different ways. For example, Brown and Harris (1978), concerned
with depression in women, studied women in a working-class district
of London. Nearly one quarter of those women who had at least one
child at home and were living in Camberwell, when interviewed at
home, showed *clinical depression*. The rates were lower if there was
no child at home, and much lower for middle-class women in Camberwell, and also for women living on the Scottish island of North Uist.
Although a *research psychiatrist* classified 62/111 of their depressed
subjects as *psychotic,* most psychiatrists consider the account to concern predominantly neurotic depression. From this study depression
is especially concentrated in certain high-risk groups within the population.

Life-time Risk of Neurosis

Is neurosis generally life long? No, but it may sometimes be. The
tendency to react in a neurotic way may be shown by a person over
a very long time and in many different situations. At follow-up of
previously treated neurotic patients, most of the subjects are considerably improved compared with their initial state at referral for
neurotic illness. One reason for this improvement is the fluctuating
nature of the condition. Initial referral for treatment occurs following
deterioration to the worst possible state, but follow-up occurs at the

whim of the researcher, and its timing does not bear any relation to the changes in severity of the patient's condition. If neurosis is cyclical to any extent at all, there may be a spurious appearance of improvement at follow-up.

In practice neurosis is not so much cyclical as reactive to what is stressful for each individual; an experience is stressful to this individual person who then reacts with a further episode of neurotic illness.

The Effects of Personality

It is tautologous to assume that because something happens to a person, that person had an underlying tendency which increased the likelihood of that event. However, some people are predisposed towards neurotic reactions to a much greater extent than others. This is variously described as neurotic personality, or disorder of personality. It remains as a life-long or at least long-term tendency. Personality and personality disorder are discussed in chapter 7. At this point it is important to consider the part that personality plays as a factor in the life-time risk from neurosis. A considerable over-simplification is represented in figure 1.4.

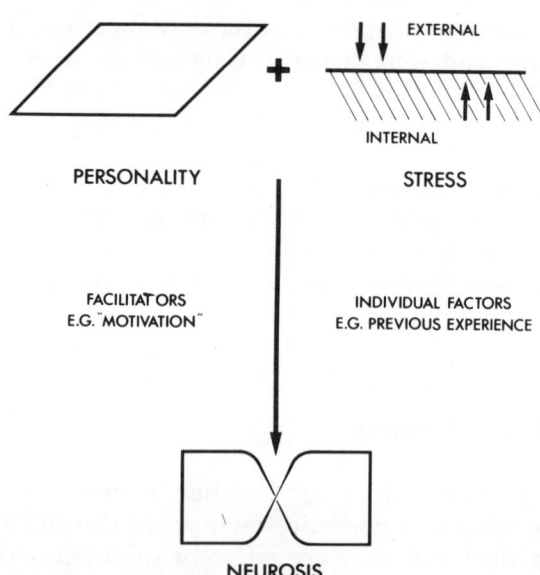

PERSONALITY   STRESS

FACILITATORS   INDIVIDUAL FACTORS
E.G. "MOTIVATION"   E.G. PREVIOUS EXPERIENCE

NEUROSIS

Figure 1.4   Formula for a neurotic reaction

Personality is always important in the development of neurosis. It depends not only on the degree but the type of abnormality. For a neurotic reaction to occur there must either be disturbance in personality or the occurrence of significant stress, or both. The greater the stress or the degree of disturbance of personality, the more likely is neurotic reaction.

A marked degree of disorder of personality with only a moderate stress or, even what to other people would not be regarded as stress at all, may result in neurosis. A Post Office sorter was promoted to Foreman after many years during which he had sorted every letter meticulously. His promotion improved his wages, but far from celebrating, on being told of his promotion all sorts of doubts and fears were raised in his mind, because of his obsessional personality. 'Will I be able to cope with the new responsibility?' 'Will I be able to do the job properly?' 'Can I cope with the strain?' 'Will I be able to get the men working with me to carry out the work to my standards?' 'Will the other foremen working with me laugh at me and think me cranky?' 'Will I be able to talk to my boss, or will I dry up and find that I cannot say anything?' As the time came for him to take up his new position he became more and more apprehensive, and finally depressed. In a state of agitation and dejection he consulted his general practitioner who put him off work with a diagnosis of depressive neurosis. An apparently minor stress associated with a very marked degree of abnormality of personality (in this case obsessional) resulted in neurosis.

Stress as Provocation

As well as the personality, the degree of stress is important in precipitating neurosis, for example what used to be called *shell shock* or *battle neurosis*. Although those with personality disorder are more prone to neurotic reaction under battle conditions, they are less likely to be exposed, as those with manifest personality disorder will have been eliminated from front line troops through selection. However, the stress of battle exposure is cumulative, and if stress continues and is severe enough almost anyone will respond in a neurotic way. The type of neurotic response depends to a large extent on individual variables. Hysterical paralysis of an arm may render the soldier incapable of continuing at the front, or the development of neurotic depression may produce apathy to the extent that he no longer cares about danger. Extreme stress, for example internment in a concentration camp, even with relatively normal personality, is likely to be followed by neurotic reaction.

One cannot leave this discussion without considering those facilitators which are responsible for the occurrence of neurosis, or its absence, in the individual case. Simply to consider the abnormality of personality, and the stress is not enough; individual factors play a very important part in whether neurosis occurs or not. A young woman with a disordered personality coped very well following her mother's death, much to the relief and surprise of those around. The abnormality of personality was marked and the stress large, but she had additional resources which enabled her to adjust to this particular stress. It is important to realise that what is stressful to one person may not be to somebody else. The Prime Minister, if she or he were asked to put the beading on top of chocolates for 40 hours a week in a factory would no doubt find this stressful; equally the operatives whose normal work this is, would find the responsibilities of government in Number 10, Downing Street, highly stressful. The individual element in stress makes it extremely difficult to evaluate and predict.

Expression of Neurosis in Different Cultures

There is a chameleon-like quality to neurosis; it takes on the colouring and texture of the background culture; it mimics physical illnesses that are prevalent in that society; it follows fashions in its presentation so that the symptoms of the followers tend to ape those of the leaders; it tends to present in such a way as to demand attention and therapeutic zeal from the person to whom it is presented. So the same individual may present his disturbances which are fundamentally unitary in nature as symptoms to the doctor, problems to the social worker, or sins to the priest.

Epidemic Neuroses

Neurotic presentation has changed over the centuries to match the changes in society which forms the background to the person's behaviour. Neurosis may spread in epidemics; it accounts for contagion amongst psychological disorders the way infection does amongst physical disorders. Although some of the epidemics of bizarre behaviour that swept Europe in the Middle Ages were undoubtedly caused by infection or by toxins, for example ergot, from mouldy corn, neurotic contagion contributed to the spread even in these outbreaks, and there were other epidemics which were probably wholly neurotic in their mediation (vide chapter 8).

Sometimes the original sufferer in an epidemic occurring in a social group has an organic illness or a psychosis. These symptoms are then mimicked unconsciously and elaborated neurotically by other members of the group. For example, neurotic mechanisms can be seen to have operated in the mass hysteria in the witch-hunt in Salem in New England at the end of the seventeenth century. How the sufferer presents his or her disturbance is greatly influenced by local expectations, and also by the theoretical stance of those called upon to treat the condition. A girl experiencing neurotic symptoms in a boarding school will not usually complain of being bewitched. Symptoms presented to a seventeenth century exorcist were quite different from those seen by the general practitioner for this girl's boarding school.

We simply do not see the large number of hysterics who flocked around Charcot in Paris in the late nineteenth century. Neither do we any longer commonly see the Victorian 'vapours'; a situation in which the lady of the house would retire to bed, successfully manipulating all those around her, whilst she reclined on her couch perhaps for years. The older accounts of neurotic illness do not describe the frustrated bevies of housebound housewives who are such a common feature of psychiatric or general practice nowadays.

Cultural Patterns

Cultural patterns and social background have their greatest influence on neurosis in the mode of presentation; whether neurosis occurs at all and its frequency of presentation depends upon other factors. Neuroses will be found amongst some individuals in any society. Behaviour may not appear to be capable of achieving the goals the individual expresses as the reason for his actions; emotional conflict in carrying out the behaviour and action inappropriate to resolve that conflict, reveal neurosis.

There are a number of culture-specific syndromes in which neurotic mechanisms appear to be important. Quite often there is also an important underlying physical cause for the syndrome. It is a feature of neurosis that it tends to build upon other existing mechanisms in causing disturbance. The person who is already functioning poorly because of some organic condition, for example influenza, alcohol excess or dementia, in trying to deal with his difficulty in coping, may use neurotic mechanisms, such as excusing his behaviour by blaming other people. The failure he feels himself to be may result in setting up a neurotic system that further inhibits his ability to perform and increases the likelihood of further neurotic reaction. Because he blamed this person he feels he cannot now ask her to help him, and gets into an argument that has further repercussions.

Neurosis itself is universal; it has the capacity to cross national and cultural boundaries, and it is communicated by contagion. The type of neurosis, the particular manifestation of the condition and even personality-type may also be culturally determined. There may be some truth in the layman's stereotype of the dour, obsessional Scot, the histrionic, emotional Italian or physical symptoms used to express misery by the Nigerian. However, the overall neurotic nature of the condition is probably present to a similar extent in each, and it is very possible that the frequency of neurosis and allied conditions does not differ so greatly in these very different cultures.

Classification of Neuroses

This section on classification follows the International Classification (1977) because this is widely used and therefore has a chance of being understood.

Neurotic Syndromes in the International Classification

In the 9th Revision of the International Classification of Diseases, neurotic disorders, personality disorders and other non-psychotic mental disorders are categorised together (I.C.D. 300–309). In table 1.2 these conditions are listed and their more important features are discussed below.

Table 1.2   Neurotic disorders, personality disorders and other non-psychotic mental disorders (I.C.D. 9)

300	Neurotic disorders
301	Personality disorders
302	Sexual deviations and disorders
303	Alcohol dependence syndrome
304	Drug dependence
305	Non-dependent abuse of drugs
306	Physiological malfunctioning arising from mental factors
307	Special symptoms or syndromes not elsewhere classified
308	Acute reaction to stress
309	Adjustment reaction

In terms of hospital practice and psychiatric referral, *neurotic disorder* is a diagnosis in common use, and *personality disorder* is common as an associated condition although less common as the primary diagnosis. *Sexual deviation, alcohol dependence* and *drug abuse* are seen quite frequently in psychiatric practice, tending to be concentrated in clinics specific for their treatment. They are only discussed in this book in so far as they overlap with other conditions. Drug and alcohol dependence is 'characterised by behavioural and other responses that always include a compulsion to take a drug (or alcohol) on a continuous or periodic basis in order to experience its psychic effects, and sometimes to avoid the discomfort of its absence'. *Non-dependent abuse of drugs* includes cases where a person, for whom no other diagnosis is possible, has come under medical care because of the maladaptive effect of a drug on which he is not dependent. Drug and alcohol abuse may be summarised as those situations in which the person shows physical dependence upon the drug with symptoms following withdrawal, or in which there are social problems arising from the abuse of the substance.

Physiological malfunction arising from mental factors is a category which is used rarely but includes various discrete physical conditions and behaviours, for example, psychogenic torticollis; air hunger, psychogenic hiccough, hyperventilation, yawning and cough; cardiac neurosis and synonyms; psychogenic pruritus; aerophagy, cyclical psychogenic vomiting and dysmenorrhoea. These conditions do not involve tissue damage and are usually mediated through the autonomic nervous system. *Special symptoms or syndromes* includes anorexia nervosa which is an important condition amongst neurotic disorders. Also included in this category are stammering, tics, some sleep and eating disorders and some other forms of behaviour more commonly associated with neurotic reactions in childhood.

Acute reaction to stress is defined as being very transient and in response to exceptional physical or mental stress, such as natural catastrophe or battle. The reaction subsides in hours or days. *Adjustment reactions* are similar reactions to stress but may be prolonged for a few months and may be related to bereavement or other forms of loss.

An Inconsistent Condition

An important characteristic of neurosis is its inconstancy; not truly cyclical but reactive, so that perceived stress from either external or internal cause is likely to result in an exacerbation of the condition. Neurosis is therefore not something permanent like brain damage which has a constant effect in impairing function. One cannot predict that all the behaviour of a neurotic person will manifest neurosis, nor that symptoms will occur all the time. Nor can one assume that improvement from neurotic symptoms will be permanent or sustained.

The nature of neurotic presentation is not consistent either. Although phobic neurosis or depersonalisation syndrome may appear to be separate conditions they may occur at different times in the same individual, or they may occur together. The different types of neurotic illness are certainly not mutually exclusive. It has often caused confusion in the study of neuroses to separate out individual types of neurosis and concentrate upon them. If this is done, that type of neurosis always seems to be more common to those studying it than to others who look at neurosis in a more general way. This is partly because of the nature of neurosis in taking on the form that receives attention, and partly because several different types of symptoms may coexist. Anxiety is commonly although not universally described by those disturbed by neurosis. Some people describe anxiety as being fundamental to all neurosis on theoretical grounds and then explain its absence in some hysterics as simply being due to its repression into the unconscious. This appears to be a circular argument.

The main emphasis of this book will be upon neurotic disorders themselves (I.C.D. 300). These are listed in table 1.3. These different neurotic disorders have in common that they are reactive but not adaptive in coping with stress; they are not in proportion to the severity of the stress; nor do they remove the threat which the stress implies. These syndromes are described in more detail in chapter 6.

An American Classification

The American Psychiatric Association set up a Task Force on Nomenclature and Statistics to produce a Third Edition of the Diagnostic and Statistical Manual (D.S.M.III, 1980). This differs quite markedly from the International Classification. Both Classifications have endeavoured to be means by which the medical profession may communicate within itself, to differentiate treatments for different conditions, and to allow comments on prognosis and aetiology.

For conditions to be included in D.S.M. III as *mental disorders* they must, in their extreme or fully developed form, be associated with either stress, disability or, in the absence of either of these, disadvantage in coping with unavoidable aspects of the environment (Spitzer *et al.*, 1978). Furthermore they are not quickly ameliorated by simple non-technical environmental manoeuvres or informative procedures, and so do not have widespread social support. (Social support would include the ways that society helps, for example, the bereaved person.) Because of these features there is an implicit assumption that something is wrong with the human organism and there is a call to the profession to develop and offer preventive or therapeutic measures. Thus *personality disorders* are included as mental disorders and are distinguished from *personality traits* which are not included. *Simple bereavement* is not considered a mental dis-

Table 1.3   Neurotic disorders; I.C.D. 9 compared with D.S.M. III

I.C.D. 9	D.S.M. III	
300.0 Anxiety States	Anxiety states: Panic disorder	300.01
	Generalised anxiety disorder	300.02
	Post traumatic stress disorders: Atypical anxiety disorder	300.00
300.1 Hysteria	Somatoform disorders: Conversion disorder	300.11
	Dissociative disorders: Psychogenic amnesia	300.12
	Psychogenic fugue	300.13
	Multiple personality	300.14
300.2 Phobic state	Anxiety disorders: Phobic disorders	300.21-29
300.3 Obsessive-compulsive disorders	Anxiety state: Obsessive compulsive disorder	300.30
300.4 Neurotic depression	Affective disorders: Other specific affective disorders Dysthymic disorder	300.40
300.5 Neurasthenia		
300.6 Depersonalisation syndrome	Dissociative disorders Depersonalisation disorder	300.60
300.7 Hypochondriasis	Somatoform disorders Hypochondriasis	300.70
300.8 Other neurotic disorders		
300.9 Unspecified		

order because it is an expected and socially supported reaction. *Antisocial behaviour* is not by itself considered sufficient evidence for the existence of mental disorder.

D.S.M. III does not have a category *Neuroses*, and so the different conditions that could be considered within the epidemiological framework of I.C.D. 9th Revision, 300-309, 'Neuroses and related disorders', are in D.S.M.III scattered amongst numerous disparate categories. D.S.M.III is compared with I.C.D. 9 in table 1.3 (above). The reason given for D.S.M.III excluding the term neuroses is that the psychoanalytic aetiological concept of neuroses implies conflict resolution by the process of symptom formation. As will be seen from our discussion of aetiology in chapter 4 the psychoanalytic concept is only one amongst many. I consider that the advantages of retaining under a collective term conditions which have much in common both in their aetiology, their course and their prognosis greatly outweighs any reservations resulting from the history of the concept. Whilst avoiding the use of neurosis as a generic term, D.S.M. III has used *anxiety state* generically to include obsessive-compulsive disorders, which may not reveal any anxiety in their symptomatology. D.S.M. III is proving a useful research tool, but it suggests a degree of diagnostic exactitude that cannot be borne out in practice.

Neurosis implies persistent behaviour beyond normality, and beyond the passing abnormalities, the short-term neurotic reactions which all people demonstrate at times. Neurosis is a repeated recourse to inappropriate behaviour involving action that does not result in the solving of problems, but only in the confounding of them and the producing of more problems. Neurosis also describes more severe reactions, going beyond the normal process of escape from unpleasant circumstances. This reinforces the belief of the neurotic that he is the prisoner of circumstances. In classifying neuroses the distinction is also made between them and *mental illness*. There is no alteration to brain processes or difference in the function of thinking, feeling and reasoning between neurosis and normal experience, but there is a radical difference in these areas between neuroses and psychoses.

If illness implies organic pathology then neurosis is not illness. If illness implies severe symptoms, disruption of functioning and potential physical consequences, then neurosis may be illness.

Neurosis from Different Perspectives

The very variable nature of the manifestation of neurosis has been described. It may mimic almost any physical illness; neurotics may be seen in all the different out-patient departments of different medical specialties presenting with symptoms but without evidence of organic disturbance. Neurosis comes within the differential diagnosis of very many syndromes, and symptom complexes. The effects of neurosis should not only be sought within those complaining of symptoms in hospital or general practice, but also in the community at large, in society, and throughout history. People carrying out actions with wide ranging consequences may not only have been influenced by subtle, machiavellian motivation; they may also have carried out their actions on the basis of neurotic thinking and decision making, and so their behaviour may have been quite inappropriate even to achieve their own goals, let alone to benefit other people.

Neurosis never affects an individual alone, relationships are always involved. It influences his family and his work. Presentation varies according to the type of agency called upon to help. Disturbance arising from neurosis is presented to the helper in such a way as to enlist his particular type of help. This is partly because neurotic disturbance really does affect many different areas of life, and partly because the neurotic person inevitably and unconsciously tries to force the helper into colluding with him in thinking that it is just in this area of life there are problems. 'If I did not have this gritty sensation in my eyes all would be well', or 'If I could be accepted on to a training course to become a typist my problems would be over'.

When the neurotic describes his own failings they are often presented as accidental rather than as something arising from any fundamental disturbance of himself and his ability to relate. So, the person with a chronic difficulty in establishing relationships describes her recent quarrel as if it was an isolated and unexpected event without causes inside herself. The danger is for the helper to look at the symptom or problem presented without considering the rest of the background. Equally dangerous for the helper is to be so absorbed by the depressing and gloomy picture of a disturbed personality that he is unable to see any way of helping.

In neurosis the presenting symptoms are often not the real problem. This is the chief reason why categorising types of neurosis is of very limited value. Various theoretical approaches have been used to explore this constant finding in neurosis that the 'real' problem is obscured by more superficial and evanescent symptoms. This idea of successive layers carries its own dilemma; is neurosis like a wheat germ with various external layers covering and concealing the thing itself?, or it is like an onion, in that when all the layers are removed there is nothing left?. This dilemma which is in part theoretical is also practical. It demonstrates the underlying philosophical difference between the psychoanalytic approach to treatment, and the behavioural; in the first it is assumed that there is some underlying, concealed cause for disturbance; in the second the symptom or maladaptive behaviour is the problem. These irreconcilable approaches will recur throughout this book, and when we come to discuss treatment, rather than subscribing to either one, we will try and hold them in balance.

Bibliography

American Psychiatric Association (1980). *Diagnostic and Statistical Manual of Mental Disorders*, 3rd edn, American Psychiatric Association, Washington, D.C.

Brown, G.W. and Harris, T. (1978). *Social Origins of Depression: A Study of Psychiatric Disorder in Women*, Tavistock Publications, London

Leighton, D.C., Harding, J.S., Macklin, B., Hughes, C.C. and Leighton, A.H. (1963). Psychiatric findings of the Stirling County Study. *Am.J.Psychiat.*, 119, 1021-1026

Shepherd, M. (1977). Beyond the layman's madness: The extent of mental disease. In: *Development in Psychiatric Research* (Ed. Tanner J.M.), Hodder & Stoughton, London

Sims, A.C.P. (1976). The consequences of severe neurosis. *Practitioner*, 216, 321-329

Spitzer, R.L., Sheehy, M. and Endicott, J. (1978). *DSM III: Guiding Principles in Psychiatric Diagnosis* (Ed. Rakoff, V.M., Stancer, H.C. and Kedward, H.B.), Macmillan, London

Srole, L. (1962). *Mental Health in the Metropolis:* Vol. 1, *The Midtown Manhattan Study*, McGraw-Hill, New York

Taylor, S.J.L.T. and Chave, S. (1964). *Mental Health and Environment*, Longmans, London

World Health Organization (1977). *International Statistical Classification of Diseases, Injuries and Causes of Death*, 9th Revision, W.H.O., Geneva

2 The Evolution of an Idea

'What the soul is, is of no concern for us to know; what it is like, what its manifestations are, is of very great importance.'

Juan Luis Vives, 1538
(De Anima et Vita)

Neurosis, like the poor, we have with us always. It has been viewed and treated in very diverse ways at different times. The terminology and the emphasis have changed in response to altered public attitudes. Theories of aetiology have oscillated between the organic and the psychological: localisation in particular organs, for example the womb, or an origin which is magical or diabolical. Theories about neurosis reflect the philosophical set of the generation which propounds them. Those disorders which we now call neuroses have sometimes been thought to originate outside the world, sometimes outside the person but inside the world, sometimes inside the body but remote from the brain, sometimes in the brain and sometimes in a 'mind' not anatomically defined. The confines of neurosis have similarly fluctuated, sometimes to include many cases of physical illness, for example asthma and epilepsy but more often a group of conditions without underlying pathology. In this chapter we look at how the term has evolved in England over the centuries.

The proponents of organic versus psychological theories sometimes took extreme measures to refute each other. King James I ordered the destruction of Reginald Scot's book *The Discoverie of Witch Craft* (1584). Scot's book attacked King James' views ascribing symptoms to the action of demons. The origins of these different theories can be traced back to Greek medical thinking where Hippocrates' approach of observation and experiment was defended against a 'theurgic' medicine in which illness, or more precisely pain, was seen as coming from the gods. Theological and magical approaches to non-organic illness gained the upper hand during the late Middle Ages, and this influenced how mental disorders were understood in England.

Much of our current understanding of the term neurosis, its relationships to stress and to personality, and its eclectic treatment methods in Britain have been influenced more by the older English medical and philosophical tradition than by European psychiatry of the late nineteenth and early twentieth centuries. The distinctively pragmatic English concept of today is historically determined by earlier writings. The term *neuroses* was introduced into the English language by Cullen (1784), an Edinburgh physician. Rowley (1788)

described neurosis amongst a variety of other conditions in his textbook of nervous diseases: 'a treatise on female, nervous, hysterical,
hypochondriacal, bilious, convulsive diseases; apoplexy and palsy;
with thoughts on madness, suicide, etc'. Two, more fundamental,
ideas for a theory of neurosis were described by Walker (1796), who
was a minister of religion and a physician. He stressed how psychological factors may cause disease and also the importance of obtaining
a detailed account of psychological aspects in the history. Following
introduction of the term by Heinroth, in 1818, psychosomatic ideas
have been discussed; for example, Fletcher (1833), was concerned
with 'the influence of the mind on the body'. In causing symptoms
of illness, 'the brain transmits the messages from the mind which
dictates its operations'.

The Mind and its Afflictions

There has been argument, especially in the earlier part of this century,
concerning the existence of the mind. I do not feel that it would be
valuable to enter into this discussion. When a practising psychiatrist
talks about the mind and mental illness, he is using it as an abstraction
which reasonably describes a certain area of the whole person; it is
not meant to be a separate part of the person, but simply viewing
that person from one particular aspect. Much fruitless discussion over
the centuries has tried to locate the soul anatomically. The emotions
and thinking processes have been located respectively in the bowels
and the diaphragm. It took a long time before the brain was accepted
to be the major organ associated with mental processes. If thinking
occurred in the brain, which part of the brain was responsible for
which function? 'There is a little kernell in the brain wherein the soul
exercises her functions more peculiarly than in the other parts' (Des-
cartes, 1650). There was also argument as to how mental disturbances
are related to disorders in various bodily organs. Hysteria was
considered to be a disorder of the uterus, the 'wandering womb' of
Hippocratic times, and this view was commonly held in the sixteenth
and early seventeenth centuries. This was the 'rational' explanation
for hysteria used by Jorden (1603) in disagreeing with King James I's
book *Daemonologie*, in which such symptoms were ascribed to
demon possession. These were two opposing theories held for the
aetiology of neurosis in the sixteenth century; the theological and
the anatomical. Jean Fernel (1497-1588) in Paris supported the
former theory although practising as a clinician. He believed that
humans were actually transformed into animals by the Devil, this

affliction being called lycanthropy (literally: wolf-man or werewolf);
a separate diagnostic category.

Paracelsus (1493-1541) achieved a rather confused amalgam of
the two opposing theories. He believed mental illnesses were *spiritual
diseases,* that is disease was due to changes of the *spiritus vitae.* He
called hysteria *chorea lasciva* and considered that it had sexual
origins. At this time hysteria was generally regarded as due to a
wandering uterus; melancholia as related to the spleen; and hypochondriasis as beginning below the costal arch.

In 1667 Willis, the neurophysiologist, displaced the cause of hysteria
upwards from the womb to 'the brain and the nervous stock' and
introduced the concept of 'nerves'. Sydenham (1681) described hysteria as occurring in one sixth of his patients. He classed as hysteria
those symptoms which could not be explained by known disease and
considered that hysteria in women was the equivalent of hypochondriasis in men (previously described by Harvey (1672) as *morbus
anglicus*). He recognised its most frequent external cause as 'from
great commotion of mind'. Sydenham's concept of hysteria was
larger than our present idea of this illness, and conformed much
more to our present day diagnosis of neurosis.

As the argument between the theologians and the anatomists
became less intense, so the need to locate functions of mind and
their disturbances in particular bodily organs became less important.
By the eighteenth century it was possible to categorise the aspects of
the disordered mind on their phenomenological rather than their supposed anatomical basis. Whytt (1765) in Edinburgh classified neurosis
into three categories: neurasthenia, hysteria and hypochondriasis.
Cullen (1784) used the term neurosis to describe 'all those preter-
natural affections of sense and motion . . . which do not depend
upon a topical affection of the organs, but upon a more general affection of the nervous system, and of those powers of the system
upon which sense and motion more especially depend'.

Gull's classical description of anorexia nervosa was published in
1868. However in 1689 Morton had described *nervous consumption*
with the triad of loss of appetite, amenorrhoea and extreme wasting
without lassitude, and earlier still (in 1669) Reynolds had described
prodigious abstinence.

The philosphical thinking of John Stuart Mill (1843) allowed a
more modern attitude towards neurosis to develop. He conceived the
working of mind with 'chemical rather than mechanical' mediation
and this allowed a more flexible and less over-simplified view of
mental functioning to evolve, and hence the development of a systematic psychology. Quantifying mental illnesses was introduced by
Thurnham (1845) in his book *Statistics of Insanity.* Psychological

causes were also investigated, for example, Carter (1853) who associated hysteria with frustrated 'sexual desire', 'amativeness . . . for the modern necessity for its entire concealment is likely to produce hysteria in a larger number of the women subject to its influence, than it would do if the state of society permitted its free expression'. He would no doubt be astonished to see the result in a society where his advice had been taken.

The confusion of the older writers on the relationship between the physical and psychological aspects of neurosis and its treatment is fully equalled by out present day confusion in this area. Neurosis is a state of mind, a description of behaviour, a psychological reaction to stress, and yet it appears to be associated with physical conditions and even possibly with an increased predisposition to death. We still think of body and mind in separate compartments despite our attempts to create an idea of treatment based on the whole person. English psychiatry today is typically eclectic and pragmatic. Perhaps here it has remained in the tradition of that great medieval English philosopher William of Ockham, who was scientifically an empiricist refusing to stretch knowledge beyond the bounds of ascertainable experience.

Springs of Action and Mechanisms of Behaviour

The first reference to unconscious motivation is ascribed to Paracelsus, 'In children the cause is imagination, based not on thinking but on perceiving, because they have heard or seen something. The reason is this: their sight and hearing are so strong that unconsciously they have fantasies about what they have seen or heard'. Stahl (1702) recognised the effect mood had on bodily functions and that this could interfere with recovery from physical illnesses. He considered that the 'life force' was responsible for all the functions of living organisms and that mental illness occurred when the soul is impeded in its free function. This inhibition 'is frequently due to a mood or, what is the same thing, to an idea which is foreign or contrary to the direction of the life force'. This was an early formulation of the unconscious origin of symptoms occurring because instinctual drives had become repressed.

Investigating the mind and factors influencing its functions was traditionally a philosophical and not a medical interest. Hutchison (1728) was prepared to 'let physicians or anatomists explain the several Motions in the Fluids or Solids of the Body, which accompany any Passion', but he himself was interested in the workings of the mind, 'we saw how impossible it is for one to judge of the degrees of happiness or misery in others, unless he knows their opinions, their Associations of Ideas, and the Degrees of their Desires and Aversions'. John Wesley advocated that doctors should be concerned with the social and psychological factors in their patients' illnesses.

The philosopher Jeremy Bentham (1817) was concerned with the mechanism of psychodynamics. He stressed the importance of 'springs of action' and 'motives', and introduced the term 'psychological dynamics'. He showed that many of our actual 'desires and motives' are unacceptable to ourselves and have to be disguised and clothed respectably by being 'ascribed to another . . . motive' by a 'sort of fig leaves'. The development of a concept of unconscious motivation in English writings long before Freud was also shown in ascribing the causation of hysteria to frustrated sexual desire.

Anton Mesmer (1734–1815) popularised 'animal magnetism', in developing the technical skills of hypnosis, which he used in the treatment of hysterical conditions in Paris. He had a vast popular following, but mesmerism produced furious controversy in the medical profession; the King of France commissioned Dr. Benjamin Franklin (1785) and others to investigate Mesmer's discovery. The terms 'hypnosis' and 'hypnotism' were introduced into English medical literature by Braid (1843), a Manchester surgeon, who investigated trance states and their clinical use.

Charcot (1825–1893) was a neurologist practising in Paris. He believed that because hysteria demonstrated observable physical signs it was therefore a physical and non-simulated condition. The fact that these people responded to hypnosis was considered as further evidence that the capacity to be hypnotised itself revealed physical abnormality. Sigmund Freud received his early experience in hypnosis from Charcot, and these ideas considerably influenced his later work. Despite the controversy surrounding its introduction hypnosis was important in directing physicians to the significance of underlying motivation and the possibility of unconscious mechanisms.

Wilhelm Griesinger (1817–1868) was in the organic tradition and a forerunner of Pavlov. He formulated the notion that psychological reactions are due to 'reflex' actions of the brain. Pavlov was a neurophysiologist working with laboratory animals. He produced, accidentally, an 'experimental neurosis' in dogs and used his conditioned reflex theories to explain their development. Followers and developers of these theories have investigated the accessibility of man and his personality to physical manipulation, sometimes conceiving all human activity in reflex or operant conditioning terms.

An early example of the application of behavioural principles in an individual case was the recognition by William Harvey (1663) of the significance of sexual factors in the aetiology of hysterical anaesthesia in a girl for whom he recommended 'hymeneal exercises'. He advised her parents 'to take her home and provide her a husband by whom, in effect, she was according to his Prognostick, and to many mens wonder, cur'd of that strange Disease'.

It would seem that most of the principles of treatment using behaviourism have in fact a long history of usage although with different terminology. For example, the method of treating obsessional thoughts by thought stopping is described by Taylor in 1660 in his account of a classical case of obsessional neurosis occurring in one, William of Oseney; the advice given to the patient as to how he should deal with his obsessional thoughts, 'we must rudely throw it away', is helpful in that it does describe what has to be done, but unhelpful in that it does not tell the patient how he should do this. It is similar in its aims, and in the dilemma of execution, to some modern methods of treatment.

People at Risk: Prone Personalities

Any one may develop mental illness, but some are more prone than others. In this section we are concerned with those circumstances which may provoke neurosis, and with those people with certain types of personality who are more liable to become neurotically disordered.

Social circumstances and cultural patterns may predispose to neurosis. In 1786 Adair, a physician in Bath, complained that 'nerves' had become fashionable. He blames the doctor who does not discuss with his patient 'what is their disease' but 'gratifies his patient with a general term'. He describes 'wretched hypochondriacs . . . who ruin their constitutions and embitter their lives, by their perpetual anxiety to preserve both'. He showed that Queen Anne's nervousness resulted in the transfer of the disease 'to all who had the least pretentions to rank with persons of fashion'.

St. Clare (1787) described epidemic hysteria amongst girls working in a Lancashire cotton mill following an incident when 'a girl put a mouse into the breast of another who had a great dread of mice, the girl was immediately thrown into a fit, and continued in it with the most violent convulsions for 24 hours'; this epidemic spread amongst the other girls.

The prevalence of mental illness in society has always been of interest and has been used in the past, as in the present, as a yardstick by contemporary prophets of gloom to demonstrate the consequences of individual and collective evil. The difficulty of measurement has long been recognised and it was realised that with a more careful search, a greater frequency of mental illness would be revealed; thus Reed, 1808, wrote, 'more people are mad than are supposed to be so. There are atoms or specs of insanity, which cannot be discerned by the naked or uneducated eye'.

In 1832 Thackrah, of Leeds, was concerned to show occupational stress as a cause of neurosis and anxiety of mind, for example, for doctors, 'Professional visits . . . afford exercise in the open air, and thus tend to invigorate health; while on the contrary, the application of mind to study and research tends to impair it'.

Abnormality of personality also predisposes to neurosis. The history of the concept of personality disorder is extremely confused, but there are two elements of personality which are emphasised to a greater or lesser extent in the different theories. First, is the importance of abnormality of personality, to what extent the personality deviates in a statistical sense from an idea of normal; the second, is the degree of antisocialness, to what extent personality influences behaviour, making it unacceptable to other people. Personality disorder is present when the abnormality of personality of the patient either causes him to suffer or other people to suffer.

The Greeks were interested in the relationship between different temperaments, the 'humours' of the body, and how these predicted behaviour. Such theories were extant through the Middle Ages; hence the physiological etymology of terms describing temperament, such as 'sanguine' and 'choleric'.

Ideas on disorder of personality developed slowly. For instance, Pinel in 1801 described 'manie sans delirie'; the situation in which the reason remained intact yet the patient was insane because his faculties of emotion and will were disturbed. Benjamin Rush (1812) believed that 'moral derangement' could occur as a congenital defect or due to disease, and John Conolly (1830) discussed the 'inequalities, weaknesses and peculiarities of the human understanding, which do not amount to insanity'. He describes the loss of the sense of proportion that occurs with neurotic thinking, 'when the impairment of (faculties of) mind is such as to superinduce an ability to perform the act of comparison . . . '. He discusses personality abnormality and its effects, 'with each peculiarity of character, will be found some peculiarity of mind, some deficiency of inequality in certain faculties'. Conolly saw a continuum from insanity via 'little weaknesses' and 'transient varieties' to normality.

The concept of 'moral insanity' was introduced by Prichard (1835). He considered this to occur among criminals who showed loss of feeling, loss of control and loss of all ethical sense, and to be equivalent to mental disease but at a different level. His views have, of course, influenced subsequent thinking on psychopathy and asocial personality disorder.

Treatments: Moral and Chemical

When organic theories of aetiology have predominated, this has logically resulted in physical, and especially chemical, methods of treatment; psychological theories of aetiology have given rise to what were called moral methods of treatment. The more perceptive physicians and laymen concerned with mental illness have realised that these two aspects are inseparable; that body and mind are unitary and that methods of treatment must encompass both. Richard Baxter (1691) who was a minister and not a doctor discussed the physical and mental elements in melancholy and 'advises all . . . to take heed of placing Religion too much in Fears, and Tears and Scruples'. His very practical approach to treatment would appear to have been more helpful to patients than the often academic and therapeutically sterile wranglings of the medical men. Earlier, in 1600, Downame, a Puritan clergyman had written his book, *Spiritual Physicke to Cure the Diseases of the Soule, arising from Superfluitie of Choller, described out of God's Word.* In this book, which is in fact an early text on psychotherapy, he described the use of silence when the patient is angry. As so often with methods of psychological treatment, the method is described a long time before any assessment of its efficacy is made. Another layman, James Howell, made the point that, 'It is true, that ther may be som distempers of the mind that proceed from those of the body, and so are curable by drugs and diets; but ther are others that are quite abstracted from all corporeall impressions, and are meerly mental; these kind of agonies are the more violent of the two, for as the one use to drive us into Fears, the other precipitate us of-time into Frensies'.

Philippe Pinel was appointed to the Bicetre in Paris during the uncertain and bloodthirsty days of the French Revolution. His immediate decision to remove the chains and fetters from the inmates initiated a revolution in psychiatry, slower in its effect than the political revolution in which he was involved, but in the long term no less significant. At almost the same time William Tuke founded the York Retreat, and initiated similarly enlightened and humane treatment in England, encouraging the individual's own efforts to reassert his powers of self-control. 'Moral treatment' actively sought to *transform* mentally ill people. The changes in public attitude to the treatment of the mentally ill was largely due to these innovators, and allowed a more benevolent assessment of the psychologically disturbed which in its turn permitted the emergence of psychotherapy. 'Non-restraint' was introduced by John Conolly (1794–1866), and he recommended the abolition of all forms of mechanical restraint in the treatment of the mentally ill.

'Moral methods of treatment' in psychiatry encompassed both what we would now think of as the therapeutic milieu and individual psychotherapy; that is, all those parts of treatment that result from a carefully organised environment in which the patient can improve, and also attention paid to the benefits of relationships, both between staff and patients, and between patient and patient. In the early years of the nineteenth century, this was regarded as an English invention, much to the disgust of Phillipe Pinel, who wrote

> 'Have the English published any new rules on the moral treatment of insanity? English physicians give themselves credit for a great superiority of skill in the moral treatment of insanity; and their numerous lunatic establishments. I have discovered no sanction to pretentions which they have no just nor exclusive claim. I have for the last 15 years paid considerable attention to the subject, and consulted all the works which have appeared upon it in the English language, as well as the reports which English travellers and physicians have published, in regard to their numerous lunatic establishments. I have discovered no secrets; but, I approve of their general principles of treatment.'

The term psychotherapy was introduced into England in 1853 by Dendy in his paper, 'Psychotherapeia, or the remedial influences of mind'. He described the 'prevention and remedy of disease by physical influence' and considered the 'pathological influence of mind . . . on the structures of the body'. There has been prolonged discussion as to which patients were appropriate for and most likely to benefit from psychotherapy. The preference for patients who were young and female was noted by Pinel in his scurrilous account of Mesmer's magnetism, 'I frequented the baquet and even magnetised at Dr. Deslon's for about two months. This resulted in a certain gallant little adventure; when my reason falls into a slumber, I am a little inclined to prescribe to the ladies the charming manoeuvre of magnetism. As to men, I repulse them harshly and send them to a drug store'. Incidentally the baquet, to which Pinel refers, was a contraption of mirrors and rods which the subjects would surround, holding hands; Mesmer would then appear with his magnetic wand, and the patients were stroked and touched and placed beside the baquet.

Group methods of treatment have an important place in the treatment of neuroses. An early example of such treatment is found in the annual report of the Directors of the Glasgow Asylum for Lunatics of 1819, 'When the patients are properly selected the advantages which they derive from their intercourse with each other, are incalculable'. Modern group psychotherapists have sometimes nominated Joseph Pratt of Boston, New England, as their founder. However, I would consider that this position is more appropriately filled by Samuel Tuke of York, writing in 1819.

> 'During the last year, I had frequent occasion to visit two Institutions for the insane, in which very opposite plans in this respect, were adopted. In one, I frequently found upwards of thirty patients in a single compartment; in the other, the number in each room rarely, if ever, exceeded ten. Here, I generally found several of the patients engaged in some useful or amusing employment. Every class seemed to form a little family; they observed each other's eccentricities with amusement or pity; they were interested in each other's welfare, and contracted attachments or aversions. In the large society, the difference of character was very striking. I could perceive no attachments, and very little observation of one another. In the midst of society, every one seemed in solitude; conversation or amusement was rarely to be observed; employment never. Each individual appeared to be pursuing his own busy cogitations; pacing with restless step from one end of the enclosure to the other, or lolling in slothful apathy upon the benches. It was evident that society could not exist in such a crowd . . . .
>
> Some persons . . . have recommended the separation of each individual instance of disease . . . . I incline to think, that the probability of recovery is greater, where a moderate number of patients associate together . . . . I incline to think the number ought in no case to exceed fifteen.'

The importance of motivation in helping neurotics was recognised by Thomas Sydenham who sent a patient suffering from dejection and low spirits to a mythical Dr. Robinson in Inverness. On return from his 'fools errand' the patient summoned Sydenham, who found his patient angry but improved. 'Good cheer' was recommended for 'the hysterical disease' by Shaw (1724) who advocated 'the juice of the grape'. Richard Baxter (1691) advised helping those who were mentally disturbed by 'pleasing them and avoiding all displeasing things, as far as lawfully can be done. If you know any lawful things that will please them in Speech, in Company, in Apparel, in Rooms, in Attendance, give it to them'.

There has always been in medicine a substantial body of opinion that regards neurotic disorders as primarily organic. These physicians were more prone to treat their patients chemically, as are their intellectual descendants in organic psychiatry. Thomas Sydenham, an enlightened physician in so many ways, yet recommended in the treatment of hysterical disorders, bleeding, purging, opiates, foetid medicines, chalybeate medicine, filings of steel in rhenish wine, plaister to the navel, hysteric julap, opening pills or electuary and many other dramatic remedies. Medicine being an eclectic practice and physicians pragmatists, a combination of chemotherapy and psychotherapy has been common; the doctor recognising that his relationship with the patient is an important determinant in the patient's improvement. For example, Valentine Greatraks anticipated exploitation of the placebo effect when, in 1666, he made his reputation by stroking the affected part of the body; he had the good sense to treat hysterical pareses and avoid organic lesions. Sedatives and stimulants have long been used. The discovery of more potent chemotherapeutic agents increased the range of possibilities, for example, John Snow (1858) introduced chloroform narcosis for the investigation and treatment of hysterical paralysis and contraction.

In the middle of the last century it was realised that neurotic patients were best separated from psychotics for treatment. Early treatment centres where less disturbed people could receive appropriate treatment were introduced. In 1860 Gaskell wrote, 'On the want of better provision for the labouring and middle classes when attacked or threatened with insanity'. He believed that 'patients should be allowed to place themselves voluntarily in treatment', and he felt 'such places offering an agreeable change of scene, quiet and retirement, as well as the benefit of good advice, would afford a means of treatment much to be desired for incipient and transient cases'. His forecast of early treatment centres of this type later resulted in many such units often associated with teaching hospitals. These units have had a particular usefulness in the treatment of neuroses.

The Stigma of Neuroses

Both sufferers from mental illness and those attempting to treat them have faced the obloquy of the medical establishment and the lay public. One physician, Cornelius Agrippa, in 1719 came very near to being burnt at the stake because of his interest in mental illness and his views concerning its treatment. Many sufferers from various types of mental illness were burnt as witches during harsher times. Although the treatment meted to societies' outcasts is now less drastic there is still considerable prejudice against all kinds of mental illness. When psychotic illnesses have been regarded as having an organic aetiology then the stigma is considerably reduced; the illness is regarded as outside the patient's control. The same excuse does not pertain for neurosis; the condition is considered generally to be the sufferer's own fault due to his inherent weakness. When more organic theories on the aetiology of neurosis have been extant, for example the physical theories of Sydenham or the behavioural theories of Pavlov, then less blame has accrued to the patient. But in general as well as having to bear his symptoms the patient has to bear the burden of shame and ostracism by his fellows. The very term neurotic, although used originally to describe a physical condition, has become a term of abuse.

The distinction between psychosis and neurosis which is fundamental to the practice of psychiatry has itself a long and varied history. Views have fluctuated from unitary theories of aetiology, to those where two entirely different types of cause are invoked. When two different theories have been in vogue, then one group of conditions has been considered to have physical aetiology, the precursor of modern psychoses, and the other type a spiritual, psychological or environmental origin, equivalent to contemporary 'neuroses'. These two different categories have demanded entirely different approaches to their treatment. Many writers, both medical and lay, recognised the need for treating psychological symptoms by psychological methods.

The stigma attached to suicide has varied very much in different cultures over the centuries, from outright condemnation to accepted behaviour in certain circumstances. The five suicides in the Old, and one in the New Testament are reported quite factually without moral comment on the behaviour itself. Amongst the Greeks and also occasionally in other cultures, for example, at Massada, suicide to maintain one's honour was accepted, although not approved by Jewish law. Ritualised institutional suicide became the custom in some societies through history, for example, Suttee in Hindu culture.

Towards the end of the Roman Empire many queried the value of existence and were contemptuous of human society. Suicide became common-place amongst the influential of Rome. This behaviour was condemned by the Christian Church as it became powerful, and in the Middle Ages public disapproval of suicide was punitive, not only towards the suicide but also his family. A distinction was made between suicide due to insanity which was not punished, and ordinary suicide which became a felony in English law. The suicide's family forfeited his goods and land, and his corpse was often mutilated; he was not allowed burial in sanctified ground.

Views on suicide gradually changed following the Renaissance. For example, both Erasmus and Montaigne were able to approve voluntary death under certain circumstances. John Donne (1608) in his defence of suicide called 'Biathanatos', wrote, 'Methinks I have the key of my prison in mine own hand, and no remedy presents itself so soone to my heart, as mine own sword'. In *The Anatomy of Melancholy* (1621) Robert Burton stresses the connection between the state of melancholy and suicide. He observes the epidemiological finding in depression; 'Tis a common calamity, a fatal end to this disease, they are condemned to a violent death, by a jury of Physicians, curiously disposed, carried headlong by their tyrannizing wills, enforced by miseries . . . .' John Sym writing in 1637 in his book *Life's Preservative against Self-Killing'* was concerned with prevention, and he considered various signs to be predictive of a suicidal attempt.

Clearly psychiatry was greatly influenced by European work from the middle of the nineteenth century. This chapter, however, shows how influential earlier English thought was in recognising the protean nature of neurosis. There is a changing pattern of symptomatology at different times and under different social conditions, as bemoaned by Adair at the pilgrimage of the nation's neurotics to Bath in the eighteenth century. We do not now commonly see the 'vapours' as described by the Victorians, nor the grosser forms of hysteria as investigated by Charcot. Earlier accounts do not seem to have had the numbers of 'housebound housewives' that are so common today. However, neurosis has always been common although different in its manifestations, and Sydenham's seventeenth century figure of one sixth of his consultations has a remarkably modern ring for the prevalence of neurosis in the population consulting a doctor. In neurosis we see a condition which has changed in its presentation and natural history surprisingly little over the centuries.

To prognosticate for such an amorphous group of conditions has always been a precarious exercise but it has been attempted over the years for, as Hippocrates has been translated, 'it is the best thing, in my opinion, for the physician to apply himself diligently to the art of foreknowing, for he who is master of this art and shows himself such among his patients, with respect to what is present, past and future declaring at the same time wherein the patient has been wanting, will give such proofs of a superior knowledge in what relates to the sick, that the generality of men will commit themselves to that physician without any manner of diffidence'.

To our study of the history of neuroses, there are some pertinent conclusions. Illnesses or symptoms occurring without organic cause have always been common amongst the patients a doctor sees. Sometimes doctors have recognised that there is no physical basis for illness; more rarely they have realised that there are psychological explanations to account for symptoms. Medical management of such conditions has divided into those who do not recognise the existence of psychogenic illness and treat symptomatically; those who realise that the origin is psychological but deliberately ignore this and treat physically or symptomatically; and those who accept psychogenesis and treat such conditions in a different way from organic illnesses.

Bibliography

Connolly, J. (1830). *An Inquiry Concerning the Indications of Insanity with Suggestions for the Better Protection and Care of the Insane*, Chapter V (Ed. Hunter, R. & Macalpine I., 1964)

Flugel, J.C. (1964). *A Hundred Years of Psychology*, 3rd edn, Gerald Duckworth, London

Graham, T.F. (1967). *Medieval Minds*, Allen & Unwin, London

Hunter, R. and Macalpine, I. (1963). *Three Hundred Years of Psychiatry*, 1535-1860, Oxford University Press, London

Leff, G. (1958). *Medieval Thought*, Penguin Books, Harmondsworth

Reeves, J.W. (1958). *Body and Mind in Western Thought*, Penguin Books, Harmondsworth

Rosen, G. (1971). History in the study of suicide. *Psychol. Med.*, 1, 267-285

Scull, A.T. (1979). Moral treatment reconsidered: some sociological comments on an episode in the history of British psychiatry. *Psychol. Med.*, 9, 421-428

Simon, B. (1978). *Mind and Madness in Ancient Greece*, Cornell University Press, Ithaca

Sims, A.C.P. (1975). The English concept of neurosis: A short historical account. *Mid. med. Rev.*, 11, 51-59

Tuke, S. (1819). *Practical Hints Concerning the Building of Wakefield Asylum*, in the Wakefield Psychiatric Museum

Veith, I. (1965). *Hysteria: The History of a Disease*, University of Chicago Press, Chicago

Walker, N. (1957). *A Short History of Psychotherapy in Theory and Practice*, Routledge and Kegan Paul, London

Wesley, John (1759). *The Journal of the Rev. John Wesley* (Ed. N. Cunnock), Kelly, London

Zilboorg, G. and Henry, G.W. (1941). *A History of Medical Psychology*, W.W Norton & Co., New York

3 An Illness that Needs Treatment

'It should seem that no chronic disease occurs so frequently as this; and that, as fevers with their attendants constitute two thirds of the diseases to which mankind are liable upon comparing them with the whole tribe of chronic distempers, so hysteric disorders, or at least such as are so called, make up half the remaining third part, that is they constitute one moiety of chronic distempers. For few women (which sex makes one half of the grown persons) excepting such as work and fare hardly, are quite free from every species of this disorder, several men also, who lead a sedentary life and study hard, are afflicted with the same . . . .

This disease is not more remarkable for its frequency, than for the numerous forms under which it appears, resembling most of the distempers wherewith mankind are afflicted . . . .'

(Thomas Sydenham, 1681)

Why is Neurosis the Concern of Doctors?

The point has been made in the first chapter that neurosis is not fundamentally organic, and therefore in one sense, not a medical condition. In the second chapter we have described the long argument between the organicists and the psychologists, and again the consensus is that neurosis is not organic. Why then are neurotics seen by doctors? Why do the medical profession, and other health professions (nursing, social work, clinical psychology), concern themselves with the management of neurosis? Professor Eysenck (1975) in his pamphlet *The Future of Psychiatry* claimed that there was no future in psychiatry for the treatment of the neuroses. He wrote, 'it seemed desirable and historically justifiable to split psychiatry into two independent parts, one concerned with organic disorders and their treatment, which in turn was largely medical in nature; the other concerned with behavioural disorders and their treatment, which in turn was largely behavioural. It was argued that the former discipline should be the prerogative of medically trained psychiatrists, while the latter should be the prerogative of non-medical psychologists trained in special courses for posts as clinical psychologists'.

This statement echoes a plea that has come from both inside medicine and outside, that doctors should concern themselves with physical illness and leave the rest to other people. It is attractive to doctors who feel more confident in dealing with organic illness. It is noticeable how much more at ease medical students are with even severely disturbed psychotic patients than with neurotics. Many general practitioners would like to concentrate on those patients who have 'real illnesses', and not deal with the others. This sentiment is also common to physicians and surgeons who are often irritated by those patients who attend their clinics without demonstrating organic pathology. There are also some psychiatrists who feel that it is worthwhile to treat the psychoses, but regard neuroses and personality disorders as wasting their professional time. Outside the medical profession there are many groups of people who would like to take over the treatment of neuroses and behavioural disturbances. In primitive societies this is often the role of the witch doctor, and where witch doctors work alongside Western-style medical practitioners, the successful witch doctor is the one who is able to spot the organically disordered or functional psychotic patient, and arrange for his rerouting to conventional medicine.

Why, therefore when they have so much other work to do, so many other demands on their time, should doctors concern themselves with neurotics? The short answer is that the neurotic will find out the doctor, and irrespective of his specialty the doctor will find himself dealing with neurotic patients whether he likes it or not. An environmental or personality problem provokes a neurotic reaction that distresses the person and he then seeks help. Where does such a person look for help in our society? The medical profession is treated as a salaried receptacle for all sorts of miseries. People with problems go to see their doctor. This importunity of patients was graphically described by Mayer-Gross, 'If you don't want to recognize neurosis as something to be treated and belonging to the field of medicine you can do this, but only under a dictatorship'.

The next reason why doctors are concerned with neurosis, whether they like it or not, is because neurotics present with physical symptoms. It is probable that neurosis is a commoner cause of vague polysystemic symptoms than those unidentifiable viruses so often blamed by doctors and patients. Only rarely is the doctor presented with an unadorned *social problem* which he is likely to refer elsewhere. Usually physical symptoms form part of the presentation, and it takes some unravelling to realise the significance of neurotic reactions, personality difficulties and environmental stresses in the causation of the patient's symptoms. By that time a therapeutic relationship has been established. A substantial proportion of the people presenting to a doctor show no organic pathology, but their symptoms can be seen as multifactorial in cause.

A 30-year-old housewife with two children complained of tiredness, a tight feeling across the face and gritty eyes. Her general practitioner diagnosed at first influenza, then glandular fever and finally decided that it was an 'unspecified viral disease'. No abnormal physical signs were found and all investigations were normal. After repeated visits to the consulting room, the doctor reluctantly asked 'if anything else was wrong'. The patient broke into tears and described her dissatisfaction with her husband whom she felt was cold and lacking in understanding and interest, and she described how she felt that she was failing as a mother and not making any friends in her neighbourhood.

The third reason why doctors and related health professionals are concerned with neurosis and need to know about it, is that it overlaps with physical illness. Neurosis is often associated with, and may in fact result in, physical illness. It often mimics physical disorders and causes problems of diagnosis, and it often complicates physical illness, so that a person has a genuine organic disorder but reacts neurotically to his disability. The two are present together and the symptoms of physical disorder cannot readily be separated from those of neurosis. A neurotic disorder may precede physical illness; the state of mind may be causative in some circumstances.

Non-organic Symptoms

The dilemma is, therefore, that doctors traditionally treat organic complaints, but some physical symptoms do not have an organic aetiology, and physical symptoms that do have organic aetiology are often associated with emotions such as fear, anxiety, depression, or enjoyment of being cared for. In the way in which they deal with these non-organic symptoms present-day physicians are the descendants of those two contending groups from the past, the *organicists* and the *psychologists*. There are only a limited number of options available for physicians when the symptoms are not organic in their cause. They may recognise the symptoms as non-organic but treat them physically, for example, a 'pain in the neck' which is treated with a cervical collar. They may not recognise the symptoms as being non-organic and treat the symptoms physically, for example, diarrhoea of non-organic cause treated with a milk free diet. They may recognise symptoms as being non-organic and treat them psychologically, for example, reassurance and some exploration of the psychosocial background for a patient with fears of cancer.

The difficulty for the physician is that he can rarely be wholly sure about the absence of organic pathology; perhaps we have omitted to look for this rare cause, carry out this special investigation; perhaps the results are falsely negative; perhaps the pathology is at too early a stage to be revealed by the crude methods of investigation available. A patient complaining of weakness, lethargy and problems coping with the circumstances of her life had been confidently labelled neurotic; her condition improved dramatically with neostigmine when it was realised that she was suffering from myasthenia gravis. One of the greatest values for the physician in studying neurosis is that he may learn to diagnose it on positive criteria rather than just by exclusion of other illness. Neurosis is a medical condition because it arrives, uninvited, on the doorstep of physicians; therefore they need to be trained to recognise it and to cope with neurotic symptoms.

In what Sense is Neurosis a Disease?

There have been many attempts to define disease and this is not the place to discuss this question in detail. However, broadly speaking, three types of definition are extant; the pathological, the operational and the biosocial.

Pathological theories consider that disease is present when there are organic changes present. However, all diseases do not show organic pathology. Illnesses, for example, moderate hypertension, may not reveal changes in terms of gross anatomical, histological or biochemical abnormality; and significant variation from normal in macroscopic or microscopic appearance or in chemical composition may, in fact, occur without illness.

An *operational* definition of disease would consider that diseases are the conditions treated by doctors, that patients are people who consult doctors, and their complaints are illness (Taylor, 1980). There are some obvious exceptions, for example, normal pregnancy and delivery, and immunisation before foreign travel. However, in practice this is a working definition that many doctors accept.

The third type of theory, the *biosocial,* has been propounded by Scadding (1959) for physical illnesses and developed by Kendell (1975) with regard to mental illness. In this theory disease carries biological disadvantage, that is, there is either an increased mortality present or decreased fecundity as a result of the condition.

Is neurosis a disease? There is no organic pathology present. However, there may be physiological changes in which neurotic patients are at the extreme end of a normal continuum; for example, hysterics in some measures of somatic anxiety. Organic pathology is not a satisfactory criterion for the definition of mental illness. Within the terms of the operational definition, neurosis is referred to and treated by doctors. This is no new phenomenon for it has been the practice through the centuries that neuroses are referred to doctors. Finally, neurosis may well show some biological disadvantage in that there is associated morbidity and probably also increased mortality.

The Nature of Medical Consultation

Medical consultation in the United Kingdom is for the patient both intimate and easy. The overwhelming majority of the population is registered with a family practitioner under the National Health Service. This registration, attending the doctor's consulting room, receiving diagnosis and prescription of treatment, and referral to specialist services is all free. A prescription charge is paid to the pharmacist, but there are almost no financial transactions between the registered patient and his Health Service doctor. As a result primary health care has very easy access, and it is personal in the sense that the patient will talk about 'my doctor', and the doctor has a feeling of responsibility for the well-being of the patients on his 'list'. Because of this accessibility, the chief constraint in general practice is allocation of time. It is not at all common for general practitioners to book patients for consultation every five minutes during a morning or evening surgery.

Human distress is pervasive and it is not limited to physical symptoms. Man is a social animal and it is normal practice when an individual is in distress to seek help from other people. Sources of help include relatives, clergy, social workers, and teachers. However, for many people the general practitioner is the most accessible person outside the family. With rehousing and greater social mobility people are often separated by many miles from their older relatives. The number of church-goers has diminished considerably over the last few decades. There is a social stigma for some people in seeing a social worker, and so those who do not feel they belong to a 'problem family' would not seek help. Obviously there are only certain groups of people who could obtain help from school teachers, and this has become more difficult with the increased size of schools.

How is it that problems which may have nothing to do with health are taken to the doctor? Feelings of distress are often associated with physical symptoms, for example, the 'lump in the throat' which occurs with misery, or the 'butterflies in the stomach' with anxiety. Frequently, patients present these physical symptoms to their doctor, as it were, as an entry ticket. The symptoms are real but they are not the main cause of the patient's distress, and to help his patient the doctor must get beyond simply considering the symptoms to find out a little about the causes of distress. What applies to doctors in this respect also applies to the other health workers who are associated in primary care with doctors, for instance health visitors and other nurses, and social workers.

When psychological or social distress has concomitant physical symptoms, the nature of these symptoms is not directly related to the psycho-social causes. For example, there is no specific bodily localisation for the distress of a person who is estranged from his wife, nor for a person who is afraid that he will be sacked. Typically these reactions or neurotic symptoms occur as a constellation, not restricted to one physical system (such as the cardio-vascular system or the neurological system), nor is it necessarily physiological in its distribution. A patient complained of sore gritty eyes and an uncomfortable feeling in the abdomen; two symptoms that had no known physiological link. Anxiety produces a variety of symptoms that are biologically related, but not all neurotic symptoms are caused by anxiety.

The general practitioner tends to base his referral of patients to specialists upon systems of the body, for example, to the neurologist or the cardiologist. As neurotic symptoms are often obscure in their origin, there is a likelihood for the general practitioner to refer his patient to the specialist in whose field the patient makes his major complaint. For example, the patient without organic illness who complains of breathlessness is likely to be seen by a respiratory physician; the person with dry prickly eyes goes to the ophthalmologist. As a result, almost all specialists in either medicine or surgery have referred to them a number of patients whose symptoms are 'functional'. Neurotics are found in considerable numbers in virtually every out-patient clinic of every specialty. General practitioners refer patients to specialists for several reasons. Those who show a problem in diagnosis are referred; the neurotic may complain of physical symptoms for which there is no obvious physical diagnosis to account for such a problem. Patients who complain a lot and are worried by their symptoms are more likely to cause their family doctor concern and he is therefore more likely to request specialist opinion. Characteristically, neurotic patients are complainers; although if they complain incessantly their doctor may come to ignore the symptoms. Neurotic patients tend to have complaints in different bodily systems, and if this is the first complaint in this system, for example the first time this patient has complained of loss of appetite or diarrhoea, then they are likely to be referred to the relevant specialist, in this case the gastroenterologist. Neurotic patients complain of symptoms at a younger age than the majority of the family doctor's adult patients, and younger patients complaining of symptoms that could point to serious illness are more likely to be referred than older.

Because of the state of our society, the services that are available, and at the same time the alienation that many people feel from their family and their cultural roots, people with neurotic problems are likely to continue to make the doctor their first source of help. If there is over the next few years an increasing number of doctors per capita of the population, a larger number of general practitioners will have a smaller number of patients on their list, and the amount of time doctors have to spend in dealing with patients with neuroses will increase. This makes it more important that they recognise neurotic problems, and treat them appropriately.

It has been recommended that there should eventually be one general practitioner for every 800 population. Many of the major acute illnesses have diminished in general practice during the professional career of the generation of practitioners who are now retiring. The major demands on the future family doctor's time will be elderly patients with multiple pathology, chronic physical conditions, and mental illness especially the neuroses. Will they give more time and attention to improve the coping of the neurotic? This probably depends upon the motivation and training of future general practitioners, which means, (i) selection of medical students who are interested in helping such people, (ii) providing a groundwork of psychiatry for medical undergraduates with an emphasis on the treatment of minor emotional disturbances, and (iii) providing further training in hospital psychiatry for all general practice trainees. There is no large scale expansion expected in the near future in the related professions of clinical psychology, social work, psychiatric nursing or occupational therapy, and so the general practitioner will undoubtedly find heavy demands made upon him.

The Relationship in Treating Illness

The general practitioner or other physician must exclude physical illness before allowing himself to make a diagnosis of neurosis, based on finding positive features. This is especially important with hysteria. The process of excluding physical illnesses may be lengthy and difficult, and whilst investigation is proceeding the patient assumes that he is physically ill. The more difficult it is and the longer it takes to make a diagnosis, the more convinced he is that his illness is serious and perhaps even lethal. This creates a dilemma in management. The more thoroughly the doctor excludes physical illness the more likely the patient is to believe that he is indeed seriously ill, and if at the end of investigation results are equivocal, psychological treatment has to proceed with these doubts in mind.

The patient/doctor relationship is one of dependence. Doctors sometimes encourage an aura of omniscience. The patient is cast in the role of supplicant; his part in this has affinities both to the child/ parent and the penitent/priest relationship. If the patient can in any way be considered to blame for his symptoms, for example, the smoker with bronchitis, then the latter type of relationship is likely. It is not only the doctor who sets this up, the patient may create it out of feelings of guilt. The doctor's habitual paraphernalia in dealing with his patients increases the feeling of authority he brings to the relationship. Taking the history and examining the patient are vital in making a diagnosis and, of course, this must precede rational treatment. However, the questioning which occurs in the history is something of an inquisitorial catechism, and, from the point of view of the relationship, the physical examination can be a ritual inter- ference with the patient's person; an intrusion which may be undig- nified. One should not ascribe excessive inner meaning to the trans- actions of the patient/doctor relationship. However, a very powerful bond is established. It is an unequal type of relationship; much more a 'child/parent' than an 'adult/adult' linkage, and the history and examination increase the authority of the doctor.

The doctor/patient relationship is also a powerful therapeutic tool. Even though it can be distorted to humiliate the patient and over- played to awe him, it has considerable potency in helping him to feel that he is being cared for by somebody who understands what is wrong with him. Whatever feelings of discomfort and insecurity are thereby engendered in the doctor, his patient to some extent wants to put him on a pedestal. This invests the doctor with superior know- ledge, and also makes him emotionally remote from his patient.

A highly competent woman during an exacerbation of her ulcer- ative colitis was referred to a psychiatrist. At interview she described her job in which she was an acknowledged expert in rearing pedigree goats, her presidency of the Woman's Institute, and involvement in the local women's cricket team. She also described her very unsatis- factory marriage; how she disliked and despised her husband but felt very guilty because he was chronically ill. At the end of what was intended to be a diagnostic interview, she said, 'Thank you very much. I have never talked so much about myself. That has been help- ful'.

Inter-disciplinary Treatment of Neurosis

So far this chapter has been about doctors and how they are called upon to treat neurotic patients. Doctors will continue to be asked to treat neurosis, and it is reasonable that they should do so. However, doctors do not have a monopoly of treatment skills, techniques or personal abilities; other related professions also have much to offer for neurotic patients, both through their professional skills and their personal attributes.

Most consultations for neurotic problems in the Health Service are initially medical, either to the general practitioner or from the general practitioner to the psychiatrist. Although most referrals come through this medical route, most treatment is carried out by other professions; the nurse, the clinical psychologist, the social worker or the occupational therapist.

For management of the patient to be planned and ultimately beneficial, the different professions need to understand what each other can do, and know what the strong points and weaknesses of their colleagues are in helping different sorts of people. For example, a clinical psychologist may well have special training in behavioural modification that is relevant for treating phobic states. This particular clinical psychologist may be a warm, sensitive young man, not obviously egocentric, and not felt to be threatening by younger female patients who have deficiencies in social skills. It is important that this member of the therapeutic team use his particular abilities for appropriate patients, and that the tougher, older consultant psychiatrist with especially keen diagnostic acumen deals with a different range of people. Ideally the different members of an inter-disciplinary team can give a variety of treatment approaches. The efficacy of the team will always depend upon the range of skills available, the nature of the individual personalities and the quality of leadership; very much less upon professional labels.

Psychogenic Illness in Hospital Settings

A proportion of patients do not suffer from organic illness but have somatic symptoms which mimic the physical illnesses treated in different specialties. Let us look at medicine and surgery, trying to assess the place of neuroses amongst referrals.

A woman aged 55 complained of pain in her breasts and was referred by her general practitioner to a surgeon who found no physical abnormality, but during the interview in out-patients the patient became very tearful. It transpired that the patient became rigid and tense in her limbs, neck and across her chest when she thought about her husband or family. She could not forgive her husband for having become alcoholic and took this as a personal affront to herself. She felt guilty that her son had left his wife and two small children and gone to South Africa with another woman. Treatment involved trying to help her unravel these complicated feelings of responsibility and guilt, and encouraging her to forgive and accept her husband. She also required antidepressant medication. She did not need surgery for her breast, and only the surgeon's percipience saved her from the knife.

In a study from Oxford (Maguire *et al.*, 1974), all the patients admitted consecutively on two medical wards were assessed for psychiatric morbidity provided they were well enough. Self-poisoning patients were excluded. Of 230 medical in-patients, 23% were considered psychiatrically ill, and 4/5 of these were considered to have symptoms of affective disorder; depression in 25 patients, anxiety in 10 patients and one patient with an alcoholic state. Two further patients were considered to show personality disorder and one suffered from alcoholism. In half of those with psychiatric illness the problems did not appear to have been detected or dealt with by the staff of the wards.

When 197 neurological in-patients were investigated in Baltimore for impaired cognitive state and emotional disturbance, a high rate of psychiatric disturbance was found (De Paulo *et al.*, 1980). Fifty per cent of patients who completed a questionnaire had scores indicating emotional disorder; this was especially likely for patients with multiple sclerosis or myasthenia gravis.

In only 10-20% of patients with hypertension is the cause known. Some studies have shown hypertensive subjects to be less neurotic than a control population. They made fewer health complaints than the average citizen; they showed lower scores for neuroticism than controls. It was considered that in hypertension a state of permanent arousal is maintained with suppressed aggression which becomes manifest in physical change (Hermann *et al.*, 1976). Situational hypertension is clearly related to stress, for example, the sudden spike of hypertension that occurs in normal students during an examination. How this relates to sustained hypertension is not known.

When 50 consecutive new referrals to a cardiac out-patient clinic were investigated (Mayou, 1973), 58% showed no significant physical cause for their symptoms, which usually included chest pain. Most of these latter did not show the more extreme symptoms of cardiac neurosis but their symptoms could be seen as 'illness behaviour'; the patient identifying himself for some reason as being ill.

When all out-patient referrals to a respiratory medicine clinic were examined (Burns and Howell, 1969), it was found that about a third of patients made complaint of respiratory symptoms — breathlessness or pain in the chest, but did not show impairment on respiratory function tests. Psychiatric assessment showed neurosis in a considerable proportion. A few had definite depressive illness, but more were suffering from anxiety or depressive neurosis.

It has been estimated that 15-20% of hospital presentations in the ophthalmological clinic are for neurosis (Karseras, 1976). In these patients no abnormality is found in the visual apparatus; when a doctor examines the eyes he can reassure the patient. A diagnosis of neurosis at this stage will prevent a long and complicated cycle of referral and investigation. First, organic pathology is excluded, then a discrepancy between physical findings and symptoms is demonstrated, and finally positive findings of neurosis are looked for, such as recent environmental stresses, or the presence of other neurotic symptoms.

Anxiety neurosis, with or without depressive features, is especially common amongst eye patients. Those symptoms grouped together under the term *asthenopia* may have psychogenic origin, with such complaints as; discomfort, aching or soreness in the eyes, pressure around the eyes, tired eyes, grittiness, chronic redness, feelings that the eyes are pushed out on stalks, tightness of the skin across the nose or pricking of the skin around the eyes. Most of these symptoms can also have an organic cause, but psychogenic origin is much more common. Sometimes a patient requests tinted glasses; these are more often required to protect a sensitive soul than sensitive eyes. Description of 'floaters in the eyes' are often evidence of psychological pathology. These spots are seen by normal people but the neurotic is more likely to complain and be referred to an ophthalmologist. Flashing lights and double vision are also sometimes complained of by neurotic patients.

Neurotic patients may also, or course, show the full range of eye diseases with organic pathology present. An ophthalmologist is at a great advantage if he can recognise his neurotic clientele, make allowances for their symptoms in his clinical examination and decide what part of his treatment needs to be for their eye condition, and what for the underlying neurosis.

It has long been known that there is an association between psychological and gynaecological symptoms. For example, high psychiatric morbidity was found following hysterectomy (Barker, 1968). However a prospective study by Gath (1980) showed that the initial high degree of psychological disturbance was reduced by operation.

It is recognised by dentists that a certain proportion of their patients have a neurotic problem which interferes with the need for dental treatment (Swallow and Shaw, 1976). This has been called dental *phobia*; fear of dentistry which is out of proportion to the demands of the situation and does not respond to reason. As these people avoid dental attention it is very difficult to know how frequent the condition is. Such individuals were found to have a profile on psychological testing very similar to anxiety neurotics. Before carrying out dentistry on these patients it is necessary to treat their anxiety.

Psychogenic dermatoses occur in people with problems in relationships or personality difficulties; usually the skin condition is produced by hand or at least aggravated in that way (Russell, 1975). Emotional influences may be mainly responsible for the skin condition, or they may be a factor in causing an exacerbation in an existing condition. Dermatoses may also be caused by drug eruptions resulting from the treatment of mental disorder, or by the use of antiseptics on the skin, or compulsive hand washing in obsessional patients. Some cases of contact eczematous dermatitis are made worse through agitation causing sweating, and scratching leading to more intimate contact between the sensitising agent and the skin. Benign skin conditions may also precipitate undue anxiety in a predisposed neurotic person.

Perhaps one of the conditions which demonstrates most clearly the blurred distinction between neurosis and normality in somatic symptoms is premenstrual tension (Tonks, 1975). Figures for prevalence vary considerably; it has been considered to be severe in 5%, and moderately severe in 16.4% of otherwise normal women. Using a postal questionnaire, premenstrual irritability was described by 19.1% of single women and over 30% of married women. Eighty per cent of a volunteer sample of women prisoners complained of premenstrual tension. In women with mental illnesses the incidence of premenstrual tension was extremely high amongst those with neuroses, whilst affective disorders showed a normal incidence, and schizophrenia a decreased incidence of symptoms. It is very difficult to decide to what extent premenstrual tension is neurotic, although the conditions do appear to be associated.

In psychiatric out-patient clinics the majority of patients referred are suffering from neurosis or personality disorders, rather than from psychotic illness. Fairly typical of psychiatric out-patient referrals was our finding that 59.6% were suffering with neuroses as the primary diagnosis, 19.1% showed depressive illness that was not neurotic in type, and 6.7% had personality disorder without concurrent neurotic illness (Sims and Salmons, 1975). Neuroses and related disorders are therefore of great importance in the psychiatric clinic, as one might expect.

It is not sufficient for hospital specialists, for example, the physician, to diagnose neurosis correctly and then refer the patient to the psychiatrist without further attention. Many of the patients the physician is treating, for example, in the diabetic clinic, show neurotic reactions to their physical illness and its treatment, as to other adverse circumstances in their life. It is important for the doctor to realise this, to continue treating the patient for his physical illness, and to deal effectively with the neurotic component of the patient's distress. The physician may reasonably seek advice from the psychiatrist on how best to carry out the psychological side of management, but it is an integral part of medical treatment, and cannot be handed over to the psychiatrist, as: 'You manage the patient's behaviour and I will look after the insulin'.

Neurosis in General Practice Patients

Most of the patients with mental disorder seen in general practice suffer from neuroses and related conditions. Watts carried out three surveys of a thousand consecutive cases seen in routine work in general practice (Watts and Watts, 1952). He tried to resolve the incidence of neuroses which had varied in previous estimates from 10% to 50% according to the 'outlook and temperament of the doctor himself'. In these surveys carried out between 1947 and 1951 psychosomatic diseases were excluded, and his estimates for psychiatric cases within all general practice cases varied from 9.9% to 13.4%. The lower rate was found during epidemics of upper respiratory tract infections in winter and spring. In a further survey of all 670 psychiatric cases seen over a period of three years, 573 cases were considered to be acute and 97 chronic. Of the acute cases, 73.5% were considered to be suffering from neuroses, whilst 52.6% of the chronic cases were suffering from neuroses and related disorders.

Paulett writing in 1956 tried to estimate the frequency of neurotic ill-health in general practice. In summarising available data at that time he considered that tonics and hypnotics accounted for 25% of all prescriptions issued by general practitioners, and vitamin, iron, and indigestion mixtures, constipation remedies and analgesics accounted for a further 35%. Many of these prescriptions were issued to patients with neurotic states.

In a meticulous study in general practice in London, Shepherd *et al.* (1966) found between one-tenth and one-fifth of first attenders to be suffering predominantly from minor, emotional disturbance. It was reported by Kessel (1960) that only 10% of those patients who had conspicuous psychiatric morbidity seen in general practice were referred to a psychiatrist during the year. The one year prevalence rate for persons with conspicuous psychiatric morbidity was 9% in general practice, whilst a further 5% had personality defects not associated with their presenting illness. Goldberg and Blackwell (1970) found that of the 20% of general practitioners' patients with conspicuous psychiatric morbidity, one-third were unrecognised as such at interview by a psychiatrically interested practitioner. It is not certainly known what are the characteristics of neurotics referred to hospital. Kessel (1963) suggests that these should be, (i) the clinical severity as judged by the degree of distress; and (ii) failure to respond to treatment.

The morbidity study from general practice carried out by the Office of Population Censuses and Surveys (1974) is a massive study involving 53 general practices in all areas of England and Wales, both urban and rural. It involved 115 general practitioners; the patient population involved was 140 346 males and 151 901 females. The actual patients consulting in 1970, the year of the study, were 88 529 males and 107 763 females. The consultation rates for neuroses per 1000, were: for all neuroses 75.5 per 1000 for males, and 162.9 for females, giving a total for both sexes of 12%. For depressive neurosis the rate was 14.6 per 1000 for males and 46.9 for females, whilst for comparison purposes, affective psychoses were 2.4 per 1000 for males and 5.6 for females. Thus the ratio of depressive neurosis to affective psychosis, for males was 6 to 1 and females 8 to 1.

Clinically there is a wide range of symptoms and of severity for neuroses in general practice. A 45-year-old manager in the engineering industry saw his firm's order book dwindling at the same time as two of his children wished to go to University. He presented in the consulting room with a tight feeling in the chest, feelings of anxiety and difficulty in getting off to sleep. A thorough physical examination and his doctor's opinion that he was physically well reassured him, and his psychological symptoms improved in a few weeks.

A single woman visited her general practitioner about twice a week for several months. She usually presented with a different trivial complaint and managed to be the last patient in the surgery, so that she had more time. Eventually in exasperation the doctor told her that she was wasting his time, and in high dudgeon she removed herself from his list to another practice. Ten months later she got herself back onto his partner's list. Over about 16 years she had been referred to five different departments of the local hospital on 18 occasions but 'no significant pathology' had ever been discovered. Her doctor had established a wary but supportive relationship with her by then which did not take an undue amount of his time, and allowed her to assume a sick role without having to demonstrate this too dramatically.

Neurosis and Physical Illness

Neurosis may mimic physical illness so that a presumed organic disease proves subsequently to be neurotic. It may complicate physical illness so that a person who is physically ill reacts neurotically to his illness, or it may obscure the presence of serious physical illness. A woman who had a long history of histrionic behaviour stole food from the other patients on the psychiatric ward. She was thought to be manifesting 'hysterical pseudodementia' but in fact had a large frontal meningioma. Sometimes a patient is diagnosed neurotic because the physical signs and laboratory investigations are negative in the early stages of a serious illness, for example, in multiple sclerosis or myasthenia gravis. In fact, with the latter condition psychiatric diagnosis has often been made before the physical weakness becomes obvious (Sneddon, 1980).

There are many areas of disputed territory. Is the condition fundamentally neurotic or organic in its aetiology? Neurotic aetiology has been proposed for asthma and various allergic conditions, in premenstrual tension, migraine and also in the early stages of more serious organic conditions such as peptic ulceration, ulcerative colitis and arteriosclerotic disease. The evidence remains meagre in favour of primarily neurotic aetiology.

This leads us to the territory of psychosomatic medicine. Is there such a thing? Is this a separate branch of medicine? What physiological processes link the emotions to pathology? Neurophysiological, endocrine and immunological theories have all been advocated.

Psychosomatic Disorder

The concept of psychosomatic medicine is most appropriately reserved to describe treatment that aims to improve the whole person; physical, mental, social and spiritual. There would seem to be nothing within psychiatry, and similarly within the whole of medicine, which is not in some sense psychosomatic; the psychological and physical aspects of illness are intricately interwoven, but the idea that psychological factors affect health directly, and induce physical illness remains unproven. Flanders Dunbar (1946) considered that certain specific personality profiles occurred with psychosomatic illnesses which included fracture, hypertension, coronary occlusion, angina, rheumatic heart disease, cardiac arrhythmias, rheumatoid arthritis and diabetes. Alexander (1952) argued that it was not personality characteristics that account for the disease, but the presence of unresolved conflict. He considered that strong negative emotion, failing to gain expression, was converted into physiological disturbance, often autonomic in nature, which resulted in physical illness. His list of psychosomatic diseases, somewhat different, included bronchial asthma, rheumatoid arthritis, ulcerative colitis, essential hypertension, neurodermatitis, thyrotoxicosis and peptic ulcer.

Let us look at some current theories linking physical illness with the mental state. These are listed in table 3.1. The 'cluster theory'

Table 3.1   Current psychosomatic theories

1. Cluster theory
2. Giving-up given-up complex
3. Adverse life events
4. Experience of loss
5. Type A behaviour pattern
6. Stress
7. Last straw hypothesis

was described by Hinkle and Wolff (1957), who have shown that illness is a state of the whole organism, 'When a human moves from a state of "health" into a state of "illness", the "illness" is likely to be manifested by a variety of syndromes appearing concurrently or consecutively, their nature being dependent upon the various factors acting upon the organism at that time'. They showed that in an apparently homogeneous sample of people, some people have a greater 'risk' of being ill than others. There are tendencies for people who have major illnesses also to have more minor illnesses, for those who have illnesses in one system to have illnesses also in other systems, for those who have somatic disease also to have emotional and psychological symptoms. Not only are illnesses concentrated within a part of the total population, they also tend to 'cluster' within a limited time for those people. Hinkle and Wolff reckoned these clusters lasted usually for 5-10 years. Unhappy experiences in childhood, difficulties in adult interpersonal relationships and heavy demands from the social environment are associated with a nonspecific susceptibility to illness of all forms. The 'clusters' occur most often when the person is having difficulty adapting to his environment. The social environment appears to have a small influence on the nature of the illness, but a major influence on its timing, the situation in which it occurs, and its course.

Engel (1967) and others have described the *giving-up given-up* complex. The person feels hopeless in the face of adversity and unable to help himself, or benefit from others helping. This complex is

closely related to *locus of control theory*; a person who has predominantly an external locus of control believes that outside circumstances control him, and that there is little he can do to alter his
destiny; with *internal locus of control* the individual considers that
he can shape his own future.

There has been considerable interest and fruitful research over the
last few years in the pathoplastic effect of adverse life events. Rahe
et al. (1967) constructed a scale for life-changes (significant life
events). They showed that both life-changes and illnesses clustered
during certain years. Illness or clusters of illnesses tended to follow
immediately after a cluster-year of life changes. The more severe
illnesses were preceded by cluster-years of higher life-change
magnitude. Some prominent adverse life events are listed in table 3.2
in the order of their significance to the person who experiences them.

Table 3.2   Adverse Life-Events (after Paykel)

1. Death of child	20. Loss of personally valuable object
2. Death of spouse	21. Law Suit
3. Jail sentence	22. Academic failure
4. Death of family member	23. Child married (not approved)
5. Spouse unfaithful	24. Break engagement
6. Major financial difficulties	25. Increased arguments with spouse
7. Business failure	26. Increased arguments with family member
8. Tired	
9. Miscarriage or still-birth	27. Increased arguments with fiancé
10. Divorce	28. Take on large loan
11. Marital separation due to argument	29. Son drafted
	30. Trouble with boss or co-worker
12. Court appearance	31. Arguments with non-resident family member
13. Unwanted pregnancy	
14. Major illness of family member	32. Move to another country
	33. Menopause
15. Unemployment for one month	34. Moderate financial difficulties
	35. Separation from significant person
16. Death of close friend	
17. Demotion	36. Take important exam
18. Major personal illness	37. Marital separation not due to argument, etc., etc.
19. Begin extramarital affair	

This work on life events has been developed by Paykel (1979). Life events are clearly of considerable research interest although it does not yet seem clear how this can be applied in treatment. It is important to realise that it is the patient's individual perception of the life event that is important, not the circumstance itself — to take an extreme example; clearly if a patient had not seen her father for 40 years and he died in a foreign town unbeknownst to her, this would not constitute an adverse life event. Life events have been studied in association with many physical illnesses, for example, glaucoma, myocardial infarction and subarachnoid haemorrhage.

As one important form of adverse life event, and as a significant predictor of illness, the experience of loss has been investigated. Various studies have linked loss with premature mortality, as, for example, the finding of Parkes *et al.* (1969) of a significantly increased risk of death in widows in the 6 months following bereavement. The recently bereaved are also at greater risk for the development of serious illness. They are more likely to feel generally unwell and seek medical help more frequently. Other losses, for example, loss of employment, have been linked to onset of illness.

There has been investigation into the behaviour-patterns of people who develop coronary heart disease. Friedman and Rosenman (1971) studied the behavioural characteristics of a large sample of normal men in California. 'Type A behaviour pattern' was characterised by competitive striving, aggressiveness, hostility and continuous working to time limits. They found that healthy subjects showing this pattern were more likely to develop ischaemic heart disease, although a number of other physical (for example, diabetes) and behavioural (for example, smoking) characteristics also predisposed.

Evidence has been collected by Selye (1956) to show the importance of stress in the causation of disease. Cannon (1957) has studied the physiological concomitants of fear and anger. The organism adapts to situations of extreme emergency by responding with a powerful emotional state which then stimulates physiological change. He described the occurrence of 'Voodoo death' in these terms.

Several accounts have seen the environmental stress of acute catastrophe as the 'last straw' phenomenon. There was found to be a high cancer rate in the following year amongst people living in Bristol whose houses were flooded compared with a similar group of people in equivalent housing who were not flooded (Bennet, 1970). It was thought that these people were probably already prone but the acute stress accelerated their illness and death.

Psychological events are not the sole precipitants in physical illness, but increasingly it is realised that illness is multifactorial and that individual stress, the way those stresses are perceived by the victim, and personality can be significant factors. 'Neurosis', in a general sense, is important in the aetiology of illness in some people. People with serious illness may react neurotically to their illness, for example, with reactive depression, and this will increase their symptoms, and may hinder recovery. Neurosis may mimic physical illness and make diagnosis very difficult.

Repeated studies according to Schwab *et al.* (1978) have shown that at least one third of all patients receiving medical care are suffering primarily from emotional and nervous disorders. The total rate of psychosomatic conditions in adult patient populations ranges from 15 to 50% depending on the type of practice, and which disorders are included as psychosomatic. Some consider that psychosomatic illnesses are more acceptable socially than other diseases, either physical or mental, that are clearly not psychosomatic.

Schwab and co-workers studied a south eastern county in the United States. This county had seen marked social and cultural changes over recent years and the aim was to see what impact this had upon the health of the community. There were 37 000 households in the county and a random sample was taken of 6.3% of these. Of the 1645 respondents 44.7% were male, 55.3% were female; 22.4% black, 77.6% white; age range 17–92, with mean age of 41 years. The age, sex and race distribution was representative of the county population. Respondents were asked the frequency of various symptoms in the preceding year. Forty seven per cent reported headaches, 39% weight difficulties, 35% indigestion and between 22 and 26% other gastrointestinal symptoms. Less than 5% indicated that they had asthma, peptic ulcer, or colitis, but 15% reported diarrhoea and 14% hypertension. These various complaints were divided into 'regularly' or 'occasionally'.

More of the younger respondents reported headache, diarrhoea or nervous stomach. More females reported headaches, constipation, nervous stomach, weight difficulties or hypertension. More blacks reported headaches, constipation, stomachache or hypertension, and more of the poor reported indigestion, constipation and hypertension. Just over 50% of the population had at least one of the symptoms or conditions regularly and 17% had two or more of these symptoms regularly. This latter group were regarded as psychosomatically ill. In this group were significantly more blacks than whites, females than males, more old than young, more of the poor than affluent respondents.

Twenty five per cent of those who rated their own physical or mental health as excellent or good reported two or more of the symptoms as occurring regularly. It appears that many people in contemporary society do not regard these psychosomatic conditions as evidence of ill-health.

Pain

Pain is a psychological experience; a subjective event in the mind. It is usually associated with tissue damage or described in physical terms, but there is not necessarily any physical change to be found. 'Pain is an exclusively personal experience, direct measurement of which is not possible and therefore the investigator assessing pain must acknowledge that his patient is reporting an experience that is subject to the influence of a variety of both personal and environmental factors' (Bond, 1976).

An association was found between personality and the ability to withstand pain. Using the Eysenck Personality Inventory those with the highest neuroticism score tolerated pain least well. This high neuroticism score does not imply the presence of a neurotic illness, but simply that such a person is more prone to develop such a disorder. An increase in the amount of anxiety is associated with greater pain. Patients with higher neuroticism scores were found to complain more of suffering from post-operative pain following cholecystectomy or surgery for peptic ulcer, and they had a greater requirement for analgesic drugs.

The typical psychogenic pain is poorly localised, described in vague terms, and without organic cause found on examination and investigation. The pain is un-anatomical in its distribution, it may have been present for many years, and investigated and treated by a variety of different methods and specialists. Often the pain occurs in areas of the body which have particular emotional significance, although it is often vague and ill-localised. Certain people with gloomy pessimistic personalities have been considered 'pain-prone persons'. These people seem to be chronically unsuccessful and unlucky, and pain occurs on the rare occasions when they achieve success. It is often very difficult to distinguish pain of psychological origin from organic causes.

Pain without organic cause in people with previous evidence of disturbance of personality may be a comment on their feeling about life in general rather than about the specific part of their body to which pain is ascribed. Pain may be, in these cases, a neurotic way of relieving conflict which removes them from some of the demands of life. Pain is very common in psychiatric patients as well as in those with physical illnesses; for example, 61% of patients in a psychiatric out-patient clinic complained of pain.

Summary

Neurosis is ubiquitous, whatever clinical practice is examined, neurosis will be conspicuous amongst the patients seen. It will make demands on the time and diagnostic acumen of the doctor. It is better for him to try and treat neurosis than to deny its existence. It is not that neurosis is exclusively medical, but the obverse of that; doctors are necessarily involved. Most of the 'mental disorder' seen by general practitioners lies within the field of neuroses and related disorders. One cannot equate mental illness in general practice with neurosis, however, as there are a few but important and time-consuming psychotic emergencies which disturb the equilibrium of the doctor's work, and are often remembered long after the neurotics are forgotten. Neurosis manifests in an enormous variety of forms and mimics many physical illnesses.

What is the connection between neurosis and physical illness? Neurosis very often presents with apparently physical symptoms. Either in general practice or in many specialist out-patient clinics an appreciable proportion of patients are found to have nothing organically wrong, but underlying psychological problems are present and these appear to have precipitated symptoms. Sometimes with quite definite physical illness, there are neurotic symptoms reactive to this illness, or arising from its consequences.

What has neurosis to do with doctors? Doctors are, for many people in our society, the most accessible source of help and reassurance, and having 'a symptom' is the necessary qualification for consulting the doctor. Neurosis is not the exclusive preserve of medicine, but the neurotic person often gravitates towards the doctor for help. Neurosis is not illness in the sense of demonstrable organic pathology but it is a form of disorder which presents to doctors, and such disorders are popularly banded together under the term 'illness'.

Medicine, of course, is not primarily a scientific discipline but an application of knowledge from many different sources to try and achieve cure or alleviation in the sufferer's state. The scientist's goal is to discover what there is and what happens. Medicine, however, is the practice of problem solving; the problem of a person with symptoms, with illness. Medicine uses science when it has applications in the treatment or management of sufferers. It has also traditionally used other non-scientific knowledge: administration in the practice of public health, the nature of the relationship between doctor and patient in family medicine. The commonly used cliché, *the medical model*, is therefore quite meaningless. There are as many models as there are types of problems to be solved.

Because neurosis presents to doctors, it is a medical problem. Medicine and hence psychiatry are defined in terms of what society at large requires the practitioners to advise upon and treat. Medicine uses science to improve its methods of treatment, and scientific methods of measurement to evaluate the efficacy of that treatment. There is nothing new about doctors treating neurosis, it has always been part of the traditional physician's role, although the names used have changed.

Bibliography

Alexander, F. (1952). *Psychosomatic Medicine: its Principles and Applications*, George Allen & Unwin, London

Barker, M.G. (1968). Psychiatric illness after hysterectomy. *Br. med. J.*, ii, 91–95

Bennett, G. (1970). Bristol floods 1968. Controlled survey of effects on health of local community disaster, *Br. med. J.*, iii, 454–458

Bond, M.R. (1976). Psychological and psychiatric aspects of pain. In: *Modern Perspectives in the Psychiatric Aspects of Surgery* (Ed. Howells, J.G.), Macmillan, London

Burns, B.H. and Howell, J.B.L. (1969). Disproportionately severe breathlessness in chronic bronchitis. *Q. J. Med.*, 38, 277–294

Cannon, W.B.(1957). 'Voodoo' death. *Psychosom. Med.*, 19, 182–190

De Paulo, J.R., Folstein, M.F. and Gordon, B. (1980). Psychiatric screening on a neurological ward. *Psychol. Med.*, 10, 125–132

Dunbar, F. (1946). *Emotions and Bodily Changes: A Survey of Literature on Psychosomatic Interrelationships*. 3rd edn, Columbia University Press, New York

Engel, G.L. (1967). A psychological setting of somatic disease: The giving up-given up complex, *Proc. R. Soc. Med.*, 60, 553–555

Eysenck, H.J. (1975). *The Future of Psychiatry*, Methuen, London

Friedman, M. and Rosenman, R.H. (1971). Type A behaviour pattern: its association with coronary heart disease. *Ann. clin. Res.*, 3, 300

Gath, D.H. (1980). In: *The Social Consequences of Psychiatric Illness* (Ed. Robins, L.N.), Brunner-Mazel

Goldberg, D.P. and Blackwell, B. (1970). Psychiatric illness in general practice. A detailed study using a new method of case identification. *Br. med. J.*, 2, 439–443

Hermann, H.J.M., Rassek, M., Schafer, N., Schmidt, T. and Von Vexküll, T. (1976). Essential hypertension. Problems, concepts and an attempted synthesis. In: *Modern Trends in Psychosomatic Medicine*, 3 (Ed. Hill, O.), Butterworths, London

Hinkle, L.E. and Wolff, H.G. (1957). The nature of man's adaptation to his total environment and the relation of this to illness. *Arch. Int. Med.*, 99, 442–460

Karseras, A.G. (1976). Psychiatric aspects of ophthalmology. In: *Modern Perspectives in the Psychiatric Aspects of Surgery* (Ed. Howells, J.G.), Macmillan, London

Kendell, R.E. (1975). The concept of disease and its implications for psychiatry. *Br. J. Psychiat.*, **127**, 305–315

Kessel, W.I.N. (1960). Psychiatric morbidity in a London general practice. *Br. J. prev. soc. Med.*, **14**, 16–22

Kessel, W.I.N. (1963). Who ought to see a psychiatrist? *Lancet*, **I**, 1092–1095

Maguire, G.P., Julier, D.L., Hawton, K.E. and Bancroft, J.H.H. (1974). Psychiatric morbidity and referral on two general medical wards. *Br. Med. J.*, **1**, 268–70

Mayou, R. (1973). Chest pain, angina pectoris and disability. *J. Psychosom. Res.*, **17**, 287–291

Merskey, H. (1976). The status of pain. In: *Modern Trends in Psychosomatic Medicine* (Ed. Hill, O.), Butterworths, London

Moffice, H.S. and Paykel, E.S. (1975). Depression in medical in-patients. *Br. J. Psychiat.*, **126**, 346–353

Office of Population Censuses and Surveys (1974). *Morbidity Statistics from General Practice*, Second National Study 1970–71, H.M.S.O., London

Parkes, C.M., Benjamin, B. and Fitzgerald, R.G. (1969). Broken heart: A statistical study of increased morbidity among widowers. *Br. med. J.*, **1**, 740–743

Paulett, J.D. (1956). Neurotic ill health: A study in general practice. *Lancet*, **II**, 37–38

Paykel, E.S. (1979). Recent life events and clinical depression. In: *Life Stress and Illness* (Ed. Gunderson, E.K. and Rahe, R.H.), C. Thomas, Springfield, Ill.

Rahe, R.H., McKean, J.D. and Arthur, R.J. (1967). A longitudinal study of life-change and illness patterns. *J. Psychosom. Res.*, **10**, 355–366

Russell, B.F. (1975). Emotional factors in skin disease. In: *Contemporary Psychiatry* (Ed. Silverstone, T. and Barraclough, B.), Headley Bros, Ashford, Kent.

Scadding, J.G. (1959). Principles of definition in medicine. *Lancet*, **i**, 323–325

Schwab, J.J., Fennell, E.B. and Warheit, G.J. (1978). The epidemiology of psychosomatic disorders. In: *Contemporary Readings in Psychopathology* (Ed. Neale J.N., Davison, G.C. and Price, K.P.), John Wiley, New York

Selye, H. (1956). *The Stress of Life*, McGraw-Hill, New York

Shepherd, M., Cooper, B., Brown, A.C. and Kalton, G.W. (1966). *Psychiatric Illness in General Practice*, Oxford University Press, London

Sims, A.C.P. and Salmons, P.H. (1975). The severity of symptoms of psychiatric out-patients: Use of the General Health Questionnaire in hospital and general practice patients. *Psychol. Med.*, **5**, 62–66

Sneddon, J. (1980). Myasthenia gravis – the difficult diagnosis. *Br. J. Psychiat.*, **136**, 92–94

Swallow, J.N. and Shaw, O. (1976). The psychiatric aspects of dentistry. In: *Modern Perspectives in the Psychiatric Aspects of Surgery* (Ed. Howells, J.G.), Macmillan, London

Sydenham, T. (1681). Epistle to Dr. Wm. Cole. In: *The Works of Thomas Sydenham* with annotation by Wallis G. 1788 London. G.G.J. and J. Robinson, W. Otridge, S. Hages and E. Newberg

Taylor, F.K. (1980). The concepts of disease. *Psychol. Med.*, **10**, 419–424

Tonks, B.M. (1975). Premenstrual tension. In: *Contemporary Psychiatry* (Ed. Silverstone, T. and Barraclough, B.), Headley Bros, Ashford, Kent

Watts, C.A.H. and Watts, B.M. (1952). *Psychiatry in General Practice*, J.M.A. Churchill, London

4 Origins of Neurotic Behaviour

'Fashion has long influenced the great and opulent in the choice of their physicians, surgeons, apothecaries and midwives; but it is not so obvious how it has influenced them also in the *choice* of their diseases. This I shall endeavour to explain. Patients are generally prompted by curiosity to enquire of their medical guide, what is their disease? But an explicit answer to the question is not always either convenient or practicable; because the doctor is sometimes ignorant of it himself; instead therefore of entering on a learned disquisition on the subject, or candidly confessing his ignorance, which would not be always consistent with good policy, he gratifies his patient by a general term, which may, or may not, be expressive of the nature of the disease. If both patient and doctor are people of fashion, this circumstance is alone sufficient to render the term fashionable . . . . The Princess, afterwards Queen Anne, often chagrinned and insulted in her former station and perplexed and harassed in the latter, was frequently subject to depression of spirits, for 'which, after the courtly physician had given it a name, they proceeded to prescribe Rawleigh's confection and pearl cordial. This circumstance was sufficient to transfer both the disease and the remedies to all who had the least pretensions to rank with persons of fashion . . . . '

James Adair, 1786

In this chapter we are concerned with the causes of neurosis. Rather than giving a comprehensive list of the myriad theories of aetiology, I will discuss just seven widely different approaches. Each theory seems convincing — for some patients, but no hypothesis explains all the facts. Those theoretical positions that explain everything are usually more like statements of belief, rather than scientific hypotheses; they can be neither proved nor disproved. However, knowledge is accumulating about the genesis of neurosis from studies of the upbringing of children, the antecedents of behaviour, and the effects of social conditions.

The study of causes of neurosis has occupied many books, even libraries, and in this short space it will only be possible to show that many different disciplines contribute to our limited understanding. Three types of factors are involved in the causation of illness; first, a provoking agent, for example, *Mycobacterium tuberculosis*, the causative organism in tuberculosis; second, a vulnerability factor which results in increased likelihood of this particular individual developing this disease, for example, an alcoholic man living in a lodging house is more likely to develop tuberculosis; third, the way the patient perceives and reacts to life crises may have significance for development of illness, for example, this tuberculous man may have become alcoholic following the breakdown of his marriage.

Genetics in Neuroses and Personality Disorders

First, I am going to discuss under aetiology the genetics of neurosis not because this is the most important aspect, but because it comes first in life. Unfortunately, genetics has become an unfashionable subject in the field of personality and human endowment, and so most of the studies are rather old. In order to separate the effects of heredity from environment, two main types of study have been devised — twin studies and family studies. In twin studies monozygotic (identical) twins are compared with dizygotic (non-identical) twins. Monozygous twins hold all their genetic material in common, that is, they are genetically identical; whilst dizygous twins, like other brothers and sisters, share 50% of their inheritance; but they do have more of their environment in common with the dizygote than with other siblings. Thus, differences in the degree of concordance (or agreement) for a characteristic between monozygous and dizygous pairs is a useful way of investigating the part genetics plays in producing that characteristic. If there were 100% concordance for monozygous twins, and 50% for dizygous (like gender), then the presence or absence of that characteristic would be wholly accounted for genetically.

Although psychosis and neurosis are not linked genetically, it has been found that when there is psychosis in a parent, there is a tendency towards neurotic reactions in the children, especially during the first two years after the onset of the parent's illness (Slater and Cowie, 1971). This would be explained environmentally rather than genetically. For neuroses and personality disorders the appropriate genetic model is a polygenic one, that is, neurosis if inherited at all is multifactorial. The genes are manifested as personality traits, and there is also a genetic contribution to the way the individual reacts to specific stresses. This relationship between genetic and enviromental factors is summarised in figure 4.1.

When the Minnesota Multiphasic Personality Inventory (MMPI) was used in genetic studies of neuroses, hypochondriacal and hysterical elements showed no significant genetic components. However the elements of anxiety, depression, obsession and schizoid withdrawal had a substantial genetic component in an adolescent sample.

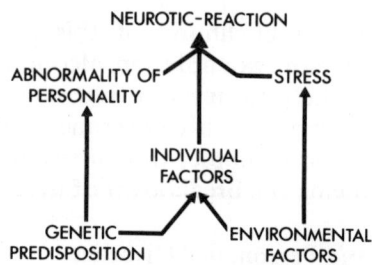

Figure 4.1   Heredity and environment in neurosis

From twin studies, there is some evidence for extraversion and introversion of personality to be partly inherited characteristics (Eysenck
and Eaves, 1979). The energy or drive a person shows also appears to
be partly genetic. When monozygotic twins were separated in early
life their personality resemblances were somewhat less than in those
brought up together. However, both monozygotic groups showed
significantly greater resemblance than dizygotic twins brought up
together. When personality measurement was carried out in first
degree relatives it was shown that same sexed pairs were more
alike; females showed a higher correlation than males; therefore
the highest resemblance in personality was between mothers and
daughters. Although environment is the major contribution to
neuroses, these findings would suggest heredity also making some
contribution.

In twin studies of neurotic patients, the personality element was
found to be of greater importance genetically than the neurosis
itself. Anxiety neurosis and the diagnostic category of personality
disorder had a marked genetic component, but this was much less
for other neuroses, especially reactive depression. When the first
degree relatives (parents, siblings and children) of sufferers with
anxiety state, hysteria and obsessional neurosis were investigated,
there was a tendency for the relatives to be suffering from the same
type of neurosis, for example, first degree relatives of obsessionals
tended to be obsessional also. For the parents or siblings of those
suffering from anxiety neurosis the incidence of anxiety neurosis is
15%. Fifty five per cent of the mothers of male patients suffering
from chronic anxiety also showed anxiety neurosis; this was the
commonest relationship to show concordance.

In looking at conditions associated with neurosis there are certain
hereditary patterns. For instance, there is an excess of both alcoholics
and teetotallers in the families of alcoholic patients. Twin studies
have shown a genetic link for the alcohol-drinking pattern in the
normal population, but there is also some evidence for genetics
accounting for their pattern of coffee drinking! There is a high inci-

dence of personality problems in the relatives of alcoholics. The genetic influence again would appear to be polygenic.

In investigating any hereditary factors in criminality, sex differences must be taken into account, as rates for most crimes are very much higher for males than females. Serious adult criminality usually starts as repeated juvenile delinquency. The environment is more important than heredity, but hereditary aspects of personality make some contribution.

Investigating the genetic bases for social attitudes, Eysenck and Eaves have found a correlation between extraversion and *tough-mindedness*. There is no simple environmental hypothesis for the origin of social attitudes, but genetic factors play an important part in determining polarisation on such variables as *radical* versus *conservatism*, and *tender-mindedness* versus *tough-mindedness*. The conviction with which a person holds his attitudes is in part genetic, and personality factors are in large part determined genetically. There is an interaction between personality and social attitudes which is also genetic. There is a lot we do not know about the effect of heredity upon attitudes of mind, personality, behavioural patterns and neuroses; methodologically sound, open-minded research should be welcomed in this field.

Early Upbringing and Child Rearing

A young married woman complained of feeling panicky when on her own at home. She felt miserable at home, spent all her time there cleaning and worrying that she might have forgotten something. Outside she was frightened of traffic, of the weather, and of the dark. She could not sit down to her meals but worried that her two children were not eating properly. She did not close any doors in case they would not open again. She was worried all the time that something might happen to her. Until her marriage 4 years before she never left her widowed mother for more than 8 or 9 hours. Her mother proved to be an anxious woman who had had a very unhappy marriage, and then suffered from a depressive illness when her alcoholic husband died. She impressed upon her daughter from early childhood always to expect the worst to happen and never to trust anybody.

Neurosis can be learnt from parents; it can also be caused by absence of, or conflict with, a parent. Some of the factors showing how family disturbances may promote neurosis are shown in figure 4.2. It is difficult to predict to what extent the child will suffer if one or both parents are absent, or if there is a lack of parental care and love during childhood, what will be the consequences in

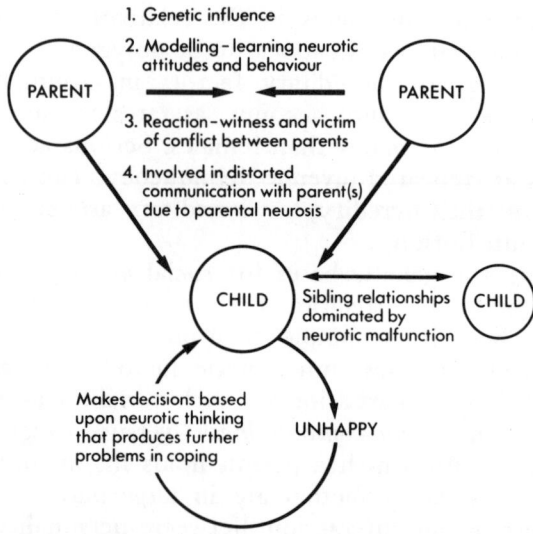

Figure 4.2   Neurotic influences upon the child of neurotic parent(s)

adult life. Bowlby (1972) and others have commented upon the extreme inportance of the bond between mother and baby established in early life, and how separation experiences are an important factor in the genesis of symptoms.

Children who have been separated from their mother in institutions, hospitals, foster homes and under other circumstances for a long time have sometimes been retarded physically, intellectually, and socially; they are more likely to suffer from physical and psychological symptoms. There is argument about whether, under these circumstances, children are damaged permanently following deprivation, or whether with a return to normal conditions they can catch up. After a time of separation from mother the child becomes emotionally detached from her. Alternatively on returning to his mother, he may react to her with hostility and be excessively demanding. The child in hospital may make cheerful but shallow attachment to any available adult, for example, a paediatric nurse, or there may be apathetic withdrawal from any emotional involvement. These latter two features are often misinterpreted as signs of good adjustment, and absence of any serious effect from separation. They are particularly pronounced when the separation has occurred during the second six months of life.

Adolescents or young adults with psychological illness frequently describe their childhood as having been disturbed; separation from mother being common, but also such disturbances as absent father, frequent parental arguments and many other instances of family misery are described. It is difficult to evaluate such accounts of disturbance made by the subject himself; his upbringing is seen through his own eyes from his present state of misery. Also, there is no adequate normative data for the emotional and psychological events occurring inside families; we do not know how much disturbance there is, and we cannot quantify conflict in 'normal', 'control' families.

The mental health of children who had suffered severe deprivation in their early years has been assessed. War orphans from the Second World War showed much subsequent disturbance, with frequent neurotic behaviour and sometimes petty criminality. Often they were apathetic, and withdrawn, describing a feeling of emptiness; sometimes they were able to make superficial social relationships, but had difficulty in sustaining deeper relationships; promiscuity was common. They often described anxiety and depression. There was some evidence of poorer intellectual performance when compared with those who had not been separated in early life. Later studies have tended to corroborate these findings, even when the separation has been less extreme, and not caused by war conditions. For example, children of one parent families are educationally behind their peers from normal families. This may not necessarily be emotional in origin; there are other factors such as less contact and teaching from the remaining parent who may have to work long hours.

Maternal deprivation occurs when there is lack of opportunity for forming attachment to a *mother figure* during the first three years of life, absence of the mother figure for more than 6 months duration during the first 3 or 4 years of life, or changing from one mother figure to another at this stage. With the increased rate of marital separation and divorce in our society deprivation during childhood is becoming increasingly frequent. The effects of deprivation are not in fact specific to the second 6 months of life. They may still occur at a later age, and loss of one or both parents through separation, of course, may occur at any age. The paternal role in deprivation has been undervalued in the past. There is evidence to suggest that delinquency is particularly associated with paternal absence.

An important point stressed by Rutter (1972) is that most experiences of childhood separation from parents are not followed by long-term problems. Where problems occur it would seem that these often arise because of family disturbances, for example, a very poor marriage relationship between the parents; this disturbance has caused both the behavioural or neurotic problems in the child and the separation of the parents resulting in loss of a parent. Antisocial behaviour in a child with an absent parent is much more likely where there has been marital conflict than when loss was caused by physical illness or death. Recurrent episodes of separation are more harmful than a single prolonged separation.

Broken homes and marital problems of the parents are significantly associated with antisocial behaviour in children, and to a lesser extent with neurosis in the children. It is the discord which is most harmful, rather than the separation, and the longer disharmony prevails the more harmful it is. Children with insecure relationships at home are also more vulnerable to psychological stress of other kinds.

It is possible that by looking at the supposed causes of emotional disorder in children, one may be able to find opportunities for prevention. Two factors in childhood which may be conducive to later disturbances are over-protectiveness of the parents and the communication to the child of their anxiety. It has been considered by Graham (1977) that it would be worthwhile to investigate the possibility of the following types of preventive action:

(1) Prevention of over-protection in children at risk. Counselling the parents of children of low birth weight or with some physical handicap about the risks of over-protection might be helpful as such children are known to be more than usually prone to emotional disorders.

(2) It is known that specific anxieties and phobias become worse if fairly rapid attempts are not made to deal with them once they occur. This is exemplified by school refusal. Education of parents and teachers, and a system of rapid identification and effective early treatment could well reduce chronic school refusal.

(3) It seems that anorexia nervosa is becoming more common in adolescence. Perhaps a change in health education, warning girls of the dangers of excessive dieting and encouraging them to seek early advice if dieting has become a problem, would be beneficial to counteract present-day education solely directed at the dangers of obesity.

Early upbringing and childhood experience is a potent factor in the later development of neurosis. Much remains to be ascertained about deprivation and the effect this has on development. At what stages in life is deprivation important? What is the minimum duration of deprivation which carries long-term consequences? Are different types of disability predominant following loss of father or mother? The cause of the separation is also important in determining whether the child reacts neurotically; for example, through death of a parent. or through divorce at the culmination of years of parental argument. What are the effects of marital discord? Under what circumstances is separation or divorce preferable from the point of view of the child's subsequent development? To be realistic a discussion of child rearing influences ends with questions rather than definite answers.

As well as the more direct effects of upbringing the atmosphere within different families exerts its own distinctive effect. This has been described by Pincus and Dare (1978) in *Secrets in the Family*. Family patterns or unmentionable 'skeletons in the cupboard' may recur through several generations.

A man aged 25 was admitted to hospital following an overdose. He was an intelligent man working as a computer programmer but since leaving his family home he had gone through a succession of disasters. He had married, had a five year old son, and had left his wife. Following a previous admission to hospital for a leg injury he had formed a liaison with a staff nurse; he wanted them to live together, and applied to the Housing Department for a flat. The immediate crisis of his overdose was precipitated by her telling him that she did not feel there was any future in the relationship.

In hospital he was petulant and demanding. At times he wanted to discharge himself. When he received a letter from the Housing Department granting him a flat he found the broken affair with his girl friend even more distressing. Reclining in an armchair in the ward, he asked to be discharged from hospital so that he could kill himself.

He had been brought up by his widowed mother to whom he was very attached, but from whom he felt he wanted to break free. At the age of 11 his father, who was then aged 30 had killed himself by attaching a tube to the exhaust of his car and had sat inside the car with the windows closed. His father had had numerous admissions to psychiatric hospital following overdoses and a diagnosis of psychopathic personality disorder had been made. A little before death he had started an affair with a nurse.

Our patient was described by his mother as being just 'like his father', and the same comment had been recorded in the case notes for the father by his mother. A pattern had developed in the family of irresponsible young men indulging in feckless, destructive behaviour which threatened to destroy the family. They felt tnemselves to be hen-pecked, smothered by anxious solicitations from their mother and prevented from 'enjoying themselves' by their wife. The only way they could break out of this was by promiscuous affairs, but once again this woman had to be protective and caring — a substitute mother. When they realised that they were trapped again in a position of destruction, they felt the only escape was in suicide. This style had developed into a family myth — a powerful explanation of behaviour within the family, not necessarily true, but felt to be binding upon subsequent generations and therefore inevitable.

Psychodynamic Aetiology

The best known attempt to unravel the genesis of neurosis by analysing disturbed processes of the mind was initiated by a person in
many ways most unlikely for such a task. Sigmund Freud found
his way into medicine, and thence psychiatry, through curiosity to
understand the riddles of the world in which we live. He entered
medicine via zoology and chemistry, and his early research interests
were in neurophysiology and neuropathology. His investigation of
the neuroses combined this innate curiosity with a need to earn his
living as a doctor, yet he considered himself lacking in genuine
medical temperament (Jones, 1962).

Freudian theory was based initially on information obtained by
hypnosis and free association from his patients. They tried to recall
the circumstances in which their symptoms first occurred. Freud
found that his patients showed resistance to remembering events
that were painful; 'repression' of these memories occurred, and they
were replaced by symptoms. Repression meant that memory for the
event itself and the emotion, usually an unpleasant emotion, associated with that event became inaccessible to conscious thought,
occupying an unconscious level, and influencing the roots of the
person's thinking and behaviour. He found that a very large number
of these significant memories were concerned with sexual experiences.
Freud believed that these sexual conflicts occurring in early childhood were essential in the aetiology of neurosis including hysteria,
anxiety and obsessional neurosis. He considered that anxiety neurosis
was caused through sexual desire being unable to reach consciousness
and gain experience in its natural form; for example, there was a
taboo against the small boy revealing or even consciously experiencing
sexual love for his mother; the emotion could only become conscious
as anxiety. Hysteria and obsessional neurosis similarly were seen as
transformation of sexual conflict into symptoms.

A married post office worker aged 48 complained of headache and
feelings of tension. He then revealed that he had recurring thoughts
that his wife was being unfaithful to him. He would repeatedly ask
her if she still loved him and questioned her minutely about her
behaviour. She was exasperated and miserable as a result. He admitted
that most of the time he knew that she was faithful to him, but he
had fantasies of her having sexual intercourse with other men. She
was more intelligent, energetic and socially competent than her husband, and he was very dependent upon her. Subsequently he talked
about his marvellous mother and how there were many similarities
between the 'two women in his life'. It did not seem too fanciful to
postulate that he had identified his wife closely with his mother. The

taboo of sexual relations with his mother had produced feelings of guilt associated with intra-marital sexual intercourse. These feelings of guilt had been projected upon his wife — so that it was she who was guilty. His psychosomatic symptoms arose from his underlying sexual conflict.

Freud claimed that these significant sexual experiences for hysteria or obsessional neurosis occurred a long time before puberty, usually at about the age of 3 or 4. Infantile sexuality and its repression were a major part of the theory for the development of the neuroses. It was realised that a sexual act need not have taken place, but experience in fantasy was just as significant in causing subsequent neurosis. Many adult female hysterics described sexual assault by their father during childhood. Freud realised that the seductions these women were describing to him had occurred in fantasy rather than actuality, but that the patient was not aware that they were fantasies; they resulted from unconscious mechanisms. The hysterical patient had experienced this sexual act (or fantasy) as unpleasant and frightening; feelings aroused caused intolerable guilt and became repressed. The patient still could not face the conflict raised by memory for the sexual act and so converted the intolerable emotion into a physical symptom; hysterical conversion.

In contrast, the supposition was that the sexual experience in childhood of the subsequent obsessional patient was performed with pleasure. Subsequently he experienced self-reproach and guilt for this enjoyment, and both the act and the associated emotions were repressed. Memory of this act could only achieve consciousness by taking on the self-punishing quality of obsessionality.

To understand Freud's views on the aetiology of the neuroses, one must realise the primacy he gave to sexual origins in infancy: 'I do not mean that the energy of the sexual instinct merely contributes to the forces supporting the morbid manifestations (symptoms), but I advisedly maintain that this contribution supplies the only constant and most important source of energy in the neurosis. The sexual life of neurotics manifests itself either exclusively, preponderantly, or partially in these symptoms'. Freud considered that amnesia resulting from repression explained why children did not recall the sexual experiences which were the foundation of their subsequent neurotic reactions. He found such behaviour as thumb sucking 'a model of the infantile sexual manifestations'.

The problem with such imaginative explanations is that they are not valid as scientific hypotheses; they can be neither proved nor disproved. If they are reformulated as (dis)provable hypotheses, psychoanalysts may reject them as not being a true representation of the theory. Such words as 'sexual' take on a technical meaning, for example, in its application to thumb sucking, which is considered to be an emotionally gratifying behaviour. Events are assumed to be happening in the unconscious, necessarily without evidence, on purely theoretical grounds, and rejection of psychoanalytic theory is in itself taken as evidence of unconscious resistance. The evidence for psychoanalysis is drawn from individual cases rather than using an epidemiological consensus. This does not of itself invalidate the theory as single case studies can be very useful. Ideally, a three stage process is required to prove a hypothesis in a single case study. First, base line measurements are carried out; then, one variable is altered with further measurement to assess the effect of that variable in producing change; finally, this is followed by a return to the original state of that variable, when there should be a return to the initial measurements. It has never been possible to carry out this procedure in investigating the claims of psychoanalysis.

Physical Determinants of Non-organic Disorder

Illness or injury may precipitate a neurotic reaction. The disability from the original illness is then partly caused directly by the disease process, and partly by the neurotic reaction to incapacity and loss engendered by the illness. Whether such a reaction occurs depends upon the nature of the illness, and the predisposition of the patient. The following characteristics of an illness are more likely to provoke neurotic reaction; an illness that is not rapidly lethal but causes long-term loss of work and energetic activity (for example, chronic bronchitis in a foundry worker); an illness that holds the threat of further deterioration or sudden catastrophe (for example, angina pectoris); an illness that makes the patient conspicuous or affects communication (facial or speech deformities); or an illness that impairs physical attractiveness or self-image (breast cancer with mastectomy).

The other important factor is predisposition. Disturbance of personality is more likely to be followed by adverse reaction to illness. For example, a person with obsessional personality, who is intolerant of any imperfections in his physical condition, is likely to react with neurosis. An athlete who used to run through the streets every morning, with a stop-watch in his hand, had a coronary thrombosis. He developed depressive neurosis which kept him off work much longer than the heart attack. Anxiety-prone individuals find physical illness to be a focus for their free floating anxiety; exacerbation of anxiety symptoms may result.

Two examples of conditions that may well be followed by neurotic reaction are myocardial ischaemia and amputation of a limb. Following a coronary thrombosis or recurrent attacks of angina an important determinant of the patient's reaction is the way he is managed by his doctor. *Cardiac neurosis* is a common condition both in those with organic heart disease and those without. Following a first coronary thrombosis the patient is sometimes encouraged to refrain from exercise by his doctor and his relatives; he is surrounded by an atmosphere of anxiety concerning his health; every twinge is interpreted as further damage; every small attempt by him to return to independence is thought by his relatives to be risky. It is therefore not surprising that he becomes anxious about his condition, preoccupied with his prognosis, despondent and apathetic. His premorbid personality is, of course, an important factor, but it will prevent a neurotic reaction if the doctor gives reasonable and consistent advice, positively encouraging a gradual return to full activity. If certain forms of behaviour do increase the risk of subsequent attacks, for example smoking, then the patient should be advised to give it up. As restricting activity does not improve the prognosis, it is best not to limit the patient in that way. I once saw an old man drop dead playing bowls. It transpired that he had come home from a wedding where he had had quite a lot to drink, changed his shoes and rushed out to play bowls with his friends. This was somewhat reckless behaviour for an old person with a previous history of myocardial infarction. However, it was a much more satisfactory way to die than anxiously waiting in an armchair for the next heart attack to occur.

Amputation also is quite often followed by a neurotic reaction. After amputation of a leg, a person suffers loss of function and disability which prevents him from carrying out his normal activities, both at work and in many of his hobbies. His feeling of deformity causes loss of self-esteem. He feels handicapped in his relationships with other people, who may avoid him and be embarrassed by his disability. He comes to feel himself outcast and unwanted. In this fertile soil neurosis may develop.

A neurotic reaction may occur secondary to physical illness and be so florid as to obscure the presence of the physical illness. Hysteria is usually a misdiagnosis when observed for the first time in a person over the age of 40. However, hysterical reaction may occur secondary to an underlying organic mental condition or a depressive illness to which the patient has reacted neurotically with illness-behaviour which increases his incapacity.

Anxiety or depressive neurosis may quite commonly occur secondary to brain disease. This is common in the slow recovery phase following head injury and also with epilepsy; it is also frequent in the early stage of Huntington's chorea. It is more common with head injury when compensation is involved (Trimble, 1981). The neurotic reactions following injury may occur as the patient realises the limitations in function he has to accept. For example, a young Army officer who sustained serious brain damage following a motor cycle accident realised over the year subsequent to his injury that he would never return to his job. This was accompanied by depressive feelings, quite understandable but severe in intensity. It is often quite difficult to decide which part of the anxiety and restlessness exhibited by an epileptic is due to the condition itself, and which is associated with a neurotic reaction to the disability and social stigmata entailed. Some types of treatment for epilepsy may also cause psychological symptoms as side-effects. Amongst treated epileptics more of their attacks may be hysterical than, in fact, epileptic (Roy, 1977).

Congenital abnormalities, failures of development and endocrine disorders are sometimes associated with neurosis. The more conspicuous is the abnormality in social situations the more likely it is to provoke a neurotic reaction, for example, a hare-lip with cleft palate unsatisfactorily treated. Late maturation, small physical size with delay in the secondary sex characteristics of changed voice and adult pubic hair, may in the male be a provoking factor for neurosis. Clearly the rest of the individual's adaptation to his social circumstances is also important in determining whether or not he becomes emotionally disturbed. Conversely girls may be disturbed by an early menarche, and the physiologically normal onset of periods and secondary sex characteristics may provoke anxiety and mild depressive reaction in a person who is unprepared, or who sees the onset of womanhood as extremely threatening perhaps because of her mother's experiences.

Stress; the Balance between Man and his Environment

One way in which illness causes neurosis to develop is via 'stress'. Experiencing illness is 'stressful'. But what is stress? Stress as a factor in the aetiology of neurosis has a lot in common with 'distress'. Stress has at least three different meanings when applied to human disorder (figure 4.3). It may refer to the response made to noxious stimuli; the person responds with an experience called stress. Stress may refer to the noxious stimulus itself; that is, this item in the external or internal environment is regarded as stressful and promotes a certain sort of reaction. Third, stress may be considered to occur when there is a lack of fit between the person and his environment (Cox, 1978).

The first type of stress is exemplified by the work of Selye (1956) who considers that 'stress is the non-specific physiological response

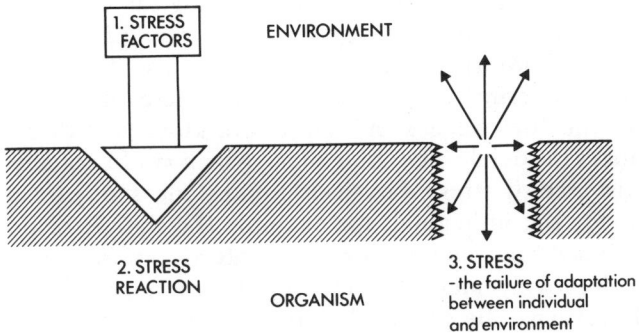

Figure 4.3   Models of stress

of the body to any demand made upon it'. So he sees certain characteristics of stress as the response to harmful stimuli. This response of stress is an universal defensive reaction, almost independent of the type of cause and almost independent of species or other variation between individuals. This he calls the General Adaption Syndrome with the distinct stages of alarm reaction, stage of resistance and collapse. These responses can result in 'diseases of adaptation', which are particularly likely to be precipitated during the stage of collapse. He considers that certain symptoms are constant as part of being ill, and independent of diagnosis. These diseases of adaptation are similar to the physical symptoms of anxiety.

Stress as stimulus implies that certain forms of provocation in the environment are stressful. These stresses provoke a neurotic reaction partly because they are intrinsically harmful, and partly because of the way they are perceived by the subject. So the extremes of sensation are stressful; for example, in terms of physical sensation, extreme heat or extreme cold is a stress, and may be a threat to survival. Where the stimulus makes excessive demands upon the person then this becomes harmful. For example, at work, either overwork or boredom are stresses. A threat rather than an actual event is stressful because it is seen as potentially harmful. This could be exemplified by the patient who receives a diagnosis of multiple sclerosis; the fear of loss of ability to function, with loss of his normal physical and social powers are clearly stresses. The problem with applying this definition of stress in research work is that one has really no idea what part of the stimulus is in fact stressful. One person may construe an experience, like parachute jumping, as exhilarating and exciting; another may find it quite terrifying. One man's stimulation is another man's stress.

In the interactional model, stress exists in the relationship between the person and his environment. This best accounts for stress as an aetiological factor in neurosis. Certain biological stages of life are especially stressful for some people, for example, puberty, the experience of childbirth, menopause and old age. There are physiological and endocrine bodily changes at these stages which can partly account for changes in adaptation. However, there are also major changes in social role taking place which could equally account for the existence of stress. Physical circumstances may be associated with stress for the individual, for example the climate or noise level. It is easy to see how such major upheavals as exposure to the front line in battle, involvement in a major catastrophe, or bitterly fought industrial action can be extremely stressful.

Family environment may provoke stress when there are circumstances such as divorce or separation within the family, bereavement or illness of a family member, arguments with siblings, or the family is in conflict with society through crime or delinquency. Stress occurs because of the way all the details of life conspire together at one particular time. Unsatisfactory relationships within the family are seen as stresses, as are problems at work like unemployment, and redundancy. In all these very variable circumstances the nature of stress is the failure in a satisfactory adaptation of the individual to his environment. Stress cannot be seen as the ultimate cause of neurosis but as system through which the neurotic reaction may be produced by circumstances.

Social Factors Promoting Neuroses

Stress predisposes to psychological illness by way of environmental factors; there is a lack of fit between the individual and his society. Important associations have been demonstrated between recent life events, and both attempted suicide and the onset of clinical depression. The use of the term depression raises the question as to whether this implies neurosis or not. As has been discussed earlier this is a difficult distinction, but where the sample of subjects for a study has been drawn from general practice or from the community at large, it is likely that the majority of those labelled 'depression' will be suffering from neurotic illness, rather than from affective psychosis.

Paykel *et al.* (1969) compared 185 depressed patients from New Haven, Connecticut, including in-patients, day-patients and out-patients, with 185 controls from the general population from which the patients came matched for age, sex, marital status, race and social class. A semi-structured interview looking for significant life events in the 6 months before illness for the depressed group (interview after treatment), and the previous 6 months for the control group was carried out. The depressed group described three times as many life events as the control group, with a significant increase of arguments with spouse, marital separation, starting new type of work or changing work conditions, serious personal illness, death or serious illness of family member, and family member leaving home in the depressed group when compared with controls.

Those life events particularly associated with the onset of depression came in three categories; 'undesirable', 'exits from the social field' and 'interpersonal difficulties'. Most of the listed life events were undesirable, but whilst desirable events occurred in both groups, undesirable were significantly associated with depression. 'Exits from the social field' implies loss of a person, for example through their death or moving away. Interpersonal difficulties were exemplified by increase in arguments or marital separation. At 9 month follow-up of this sample, those depressesd patients who had recovered showed fewer exits and fewer undesirable life events in the previous 6 months than those previously depressed who had not recovered. It was considered that adverse life events were significantly associated with the onset of depression.

Brown and Harris (1978) described the social origins of depression. A large sample of women living in Camberwell were interviewed; 15% were considered to have suffered from a definite affective disorder during the three previous months. These women were thought to be suffering from symptoms of such severity that they would have received a psychiatric diagnosis if they had been referred to out-patients. A further 18% of women were suffering from borderline conditions; that is they had definite psychiatric symptoms which were not considered to be severe enough to rate as 'cases'. Depression was very common among working class women in London, but not amongst women in a rural population in the Outer Hebrides. When they investigated causes they described provoking agents which decided the time when the depression occurred, vulnerability factors which predicted whether these provoking agents would have an effect, and symptom formation factors which determined the severity and form of the depressive illness.

It was the way she saw the changes in her life, rather than the changes themselves that were crucial for determing depression. It was therefore not the life event or provoking agent alone which was important but the meaning of the event to the individual, and especially those events with longer term implications. Characteristic of the way vulnerablility factors worked on the provoking agents would be the case of a working class woman with children but no husband; there was no one at home in whom she could confide. She was, then, more likely to break down in the presence of a severe life event. Similarly having three or more children under the age of 14 at home, or having lost her mother before the age of 11, increases the risk in the presence of a provoking agent. The study of life events and social origins in depression holds considerable hope for establishing rational bases for treatment.

Learning Theory and the Development of Neurosis

Reactive depression is a synonym for depressive neurosis. We have discussed how it may well have social origins; other models also repay investigation. The sufferer usually describes a feeling of helplessness. This experience of helplessness is also linked with the 'giving-up given-up complex', which has been described in the early stages of severe physical illness, and is rather similar to the 'adaptation syndrome' of Selye. Seligman and Maier (1967), and Miller and Seligman (1975), elaborating experimental procedures used in animals, have developed the concept of *learned helplessness*. A dog is given electric shocks in a shuttle box. It runs frantically about and accidently escapes over the barrier. On repeating this procedure it learns to escape more quickly. If dogs are regularly given shocks from which they cannot escape and then placed in this shuttle box, they do not try to escape but passively accept the shocks. This reaction to the impossibility of escape from an harmful stimulus is called *learned helplessness*.

This model was applied to human depression in which it was considered that the patient had learned to accept the vicissitudes of his environment with helplessness rather than with any attempt to overcome his difficulties. The corollary of course is that treatment involves learning that he is not as helpless as he thought he was; and that he can become an effective human being and alter his environment, at least to some extent.

Learned helplessness is one behavioural theory for the origin of depression. Behavioural models have been produced for other areas of neurotic behaviour, for example, the manifestation of anxiety and phobic symptoms. Two theories for the learning of symptoms will be mentioned here briefly. The first is the classical Pavlovian model of conditioning (Pavlov, 1927). An unconditional stimulus is followed by an appropriate response (food placed in the mouth is followed by salivation). If a conditional stimulus is then repeatedly presented just before the unconditional stimulus, the response will eventually be produced by the conditional stimulus alone (regularly shining a light before presentation of food will produce salivation with just the light). If the conditional stimulus is no longer paired with the unconditional stimulus, extinction of the conditional response eventually occurs (salivation on shining the light no longer happens).

It has been postulated that neurotic behaviour may develop according to the principles of conditioning. The neurotic behaviour is seen as a learnt response in which a conditional stimulus provokes an inappropriate response to anxiety. This was first described by Pavlov when a flood nearly drowned, and absolutely terrified, his dogs in the animal house in Leningrad. Water, in small amounts, became for some animals a conditional stimulus with the response of panic.

In classical conditioning then, a conditioned stimulus results in the response of neurotic behaviour. For example, if sexual interest as a child is always punished, that person when adult may come to associate fear and anxiety with sexual arousal, with resultant conflict. However this single model does not really fit neurosis in humans. Reinforcement is required to produce a conditioned response; that is, the unconditional stimulus must follow the conditional stimulus repeatedly; otherwise extinction will occur, with loss of the reflex.

This has been explained on the basis that some neurotic behaviours do not seem to be subject to the laws of extinction (Eysenck, 1976). The concept of incubation is invoked which means that responses that do not extinguish in the presence of the conditional stimulus alone are ones where the underlying anxiety or fear response is enhanced. The responses that are most likely to be enhanced are those where the conditional stimulus has acquired 'drive' properties. Other factors that might contribute to incubation are personality traits and length of presentation of the conditional stimulus.

Operant conditioning was a term introduced by Skinner (1938). Operant behaviour is a voluntary response to a discriminative stimulus; choosing what we will do, which choice we will make, in response to circumstances. Food placed before a hungry man stimulates salivation irrespective of whether he wishes it. If the telephone rings we may choose to answer it or ignore it — that is the telephone is a discriminative stimulus and answering it is operant behaviour. Operant conditioning works on the principle of rewards or reinforcers; we answer the telephone hoping that it will be somebody we want to talk to. Theories for the aetiology of neuroses have been based on this form of learning — that the neurotic behaviour is learnt by reinforcement.

One of the easiest situations in which to see operant conditioning causative in neurosis is in addictive behaviour. For example, although many may enjoy an occasional game, a few people become 'hooked' on a one-arm bandit or electronic game. Success gives partial reinforcements, that is for many attempts there is only occasional reward but this reward is enough to maintain the behaviour. Again, this simple model is insufficient on its own to explain the complexities of neurotic behaviour, but it has some usefulness in indicating possible methods of treatment.

Animal models have been used extensively for investigating the causes of neurosis. Hebb (1947), for example, has listed six criteria for defining neurosis in animals: It is (1) undesirable, (2) emotional, (3) generalised, (4) persistent or chronic, (5) statistically abnormal, and (6) not caused by a specific gross neural lesion. However these criteria are not specific to neurosis. They could, for example, all describe some of the vagaries of the human animal's behaviour not normally regarded as neurotic, such as involvement in minority extreme politics. So far animal work has illuminated the origins of some symptoms but has not made a direct contribution to the understanding of human neurosis in general.

There is no single cause of neurosis. Neither can any one theoretical standpoint or model wholly satisfy us in explaining all neurotic reactions. All the different theories described seem to have validity in some situations. It is not events that cause neurosis but the individual's perception and interpretation of those events; what they mean to him and how they signify changes or inevitability in his life. 'The source of neurotic disorder lies in the situations and conflicts which engage the individual in his world and which only become crucial because of specific mechanisms that lead to certain transformations of experience not normally found' (Jaspers, 1963).

Bibliography

Adair, J. (1786). *Medical Cautions for the Consideration of Invalids; those Especially who Resort to Bath*, Dodsley & Dilly, Bath

Bowlby, J. (1972). *Child Care and the Growth of Love*, 2nd edn, Penguin Books, London

Brown, G.W. and Harris, T. (1978). *Social Origins of Depression*, Tavistock Publications, London

Cox, T. (1978). *Stress*, Macmillan, London

Eysenck, H.J. (1976). The learning theory model of neurosis – a new approach. *Behav. Res. Ther.*, 14, 251–267

Eysenck, H.J. and Eaves, L. (1979). A genetic basis for social attitudes? In: *Psychiatry, Genetics and Pathography* (Ed. Roth, M. and Cowie, V.), Gaskell Press, London

Freud, S. (1938). Three contributions to the theory of sex. In: *The Basic Writings of Sigmund Freud* (Ed. and trans. by A.A. Brill), The Modern Way, New York

Graham, P.J. (1977). *Epidemiological Approaches in Child Psychiatry*, Academic Press, London

Hebb, D.O. (1947). Spontaneous neurosis in chimpanzees: Theoretical relations with clinical and experimental phenomena. *Psychosom. Med.*, 9, 3–16

Jaspers, K. (1963). *General Psychopathology*, 7th edn, (Trans. Hoenig, J. and Hamilton, M.W.), Manchester University Press

Jones, E. (1962). *The Life and Work of Sigmund Freud*, Pelican Books, Harmondsworth

Maser, J.D. and Seligman, M.E.P. (1977). *Psychopathology: Experimental Models*, W.H. Freeman, San Francisco

Miller, W.R. and Seligman, M.E.P. (1975). Depression and learned helplessness in man. *J. Abn. Psychol.*, **84**, 228–238

Pavlov, I.P. (1927). *Conditioned Reflexes*, Oxford, Oxford University Press

Paykel, E.S., Myers, J.K., Dienelt, M.N., Klerman, G.L., Lindenthal, J.J. and Pepper, M.P. (1969). Life events and depression: A controlled study. *Arch. gen. Psychiat.*, **21**, 753–760

Pincus, L. and Dare, C. (1978). *Secrets in the Family*, Faber & Faber, Boston

Roy, A. (1977). Identification and hysterical symptoms. *Br. J. med. Psychol.*, **50**, 317–318

Rutter, M. (1972). *Maternal Deprivation Reassessed*, Penguin Books, Harmondsworth

Seligman, M.E.P. and Maier, S.F. (1967). Failure to escape traumatic shock. *J. exp. Psychol.*, **74**, 1–9

Selye, H. (1956). *The Stress of Life*, McGraw-Hill, New York

Skinner, B.F. (1938). *The Behaviour of Organisms*, Appleton-Century-Crofts, New York

Slater, E. and Cowie, V. (1971). *The Genetics of Mental Disorders*, Oxford University Press, London

Trimble, M.R. (1981). *Post-traumatic Neurosis: From Railway Spine to the Whiplash*, John Wiley, Chichester

5   Course, Outcome and its Evaluation

'People never die of love or grief alone; though some die of inherent maladies, which the tortures of those passions prematurely force into destructive action'.

Charlotte Bronte: 'Shirley', 1849

In order to study the course and outcome of neurosis, the principles of epidemiology as they apply to psychiatry become relevant. These have been described and helpful applications demonstrated by Hare and Wing (1970), and by Cooper and Morgan (1973). The essential elements of choosing an appropriate population sample and carrying out a meaningful survey have been discussed by Moser and Kalton (1971). Epidemiological work with the neuroses is extremely difficult; it is rather like sculpting in butter — a very slight change in the climate and one is presented with a totally meaningless mess.

Natural History

In using the term natural history about neurosis I am really making three assertions. First, that neurotic illnesses have enough features in common to be considered an entity; second, that a common course for these conditions can be charted; third, this course can be affected by major events, but without these a more or less predictable, or natural outcome will ensue. Greer and Cawley (1966) have considered, in the context of neurotic disorders, that natural history could be defined as 'the development of clinical features, social events, course and outcome of an illness'. In this chapter we are particularly concerned with the course and outcome.

Neurosis can last a long time; to assess the natural history it is necessary to observe and record the clinical features of the same large number of neurotic patients at different times. For this reason follow-up studies are essential for neurosis, to ascertain the likely course and prognosis. The late Dr P.D. Scott said, 'The follow-up is the great exposer of truth, the rock on which many fine theories are wrecked and upon which better ones can be built; it is to the psychiatrist what the post mortem is to the physician' (1969).

Considerable caution is required in accepting statements on the natural history of neurosis; the first and most important requirement is to look at the population on which the study was performed. For example, the outcome of a psychiatric in-patient population will be quite different from that of neurotic patients diagnosed in general practice, and both will differ markedly from that of neurotic reactions seen in a prison population. We have already discussed the differences between the more severely disturbed neurotic person seen in hospital, and the larger number of less disturbed people in general practice. Do they have other differences between them apart from the severity of their neurosis? The answer to this question is almost certainly, yes.

The follow-up of a number of people with neurotic disorders will fill in many gaps in our knowledge. It should not be seen as conflicting with the detailed study of individual patients, for example, psychodynamic explanations for their symptoms; the two approaches are complementary. One also wants to know what happens to people with symptoms who are not treated, so that one can compare this with the results of those who are. It is important to assess the effects of different sorts of treatments, and it is also important to look at the differing outcomes of the various presentations and symptoms of the neuroses.

I have attempted to answer in the third chapter whether neurosis is illness. The natural history of neurosis also demonstrates some of the characteristics of illness. Is it legitimate to talk about neurosis as a single condition? Are not the differences between different types of neurosis so great that they must be considered separately? This is a reasonable question, but when considering outcome, the similarities between different neurotic syndromes outweigh their differences. The most satisfactory approach is to consider the natural history of all neuroses, and then to see whether the sub-groups behave differently.

Course and Outcome

Because neurosis is so ill-defined as a condition, there is some confusion about prognosis. What we do know about neurosis has been gleaned from follow-up studies with large numbers of patients, to neutralise environmental and other factors affecting the course and outcome in any given individual.

In practice, psychiatrists are reasonably accurate at predicting the outcome of their patients' illness. This was suggested by two findings. First, the prognosis recorded by psychiatrists in the case notes at the time of discharge of neurotic patients was found to predict significantly actual outcome at 12 year follow-up. Second, when three psychiatrists, who worked independently, were asked to rate prognosis for a group of 40 patients after reading detailed case summaries,

their predictions for outcome for these patients correlated significantly with each other, and with the actual outcome assessed at
follow-up interview (Sims, 1974).

Age of Onset

Usually neurosis is first recognised in young adults. However, such
people will often have shown neurotic traits in adolescence, and have
been predisposed to early adult neurotic illness both by personality
and by upbringing and family background. The first instance of
neurotic illness is usually precipitated by environmental stress. It is
common for such precipitants to involve situations in which the
patient has failed in personal relationships at work, or in his marriage
or family. Early adult life is associated with many major life changes,
and it is often one or several of these that act as the trigger for neurotic
reaction.

Neurosis always has for the individual large scale social implications.
In early adult life these are particularly critical. This is the stage
when decisions are made, about marriage and work and future life
goals and attitudes, that affect the whole of the rest of one's life. If
these decisions are influenced by neurotic thinking, the subsequent
quality of that person's life may be impaired substantially.

A girl student shared a house with five men, one of whom, ten
years older than herself, was her lover. She was very unhappy, felt
herself unable to make relationships, and believed that she was
unattractive and abnormal, although actually well-favoured. She clung
to her boyfriend because he took notice of her. At the same time he
was also often very cruel, making disparaging remarks about her
figure and telling her about his numerous amorous affairs with other
girls. She could not bring herself to leave him because of her feelings
of inadequacy; her attachment was sustained for neurotic reasons.
When eventually this affair broke up, it was followed by a succession
of casual liaisons with men who could not for various reasons make a
lasting relationship with her. She said of herself that after her first
affair she could not feel a real person unless she was living with a
man and yet could only choose people who abused and finally
abandoned her.

Although the first episode of neurotic illness coming to professional
attention is commonly in early life, neurotic reactions can occur at
any age. Those occurring at a later age are especially likely to be
provoked by physical illness or by the experience of loss. A person
who has responded neurotically at one time of stress is more likely
to show neurotic reactions subsequently.

Course through Life

It is very difficult to predict the likely course through life of the neurotic; to ascertain whether he is likely to be improved, the same or worse when seen on subsequent occasions. Several hundred follow-up studies of neurosis have been carried out since Grant (1925) described the course of 865 British soldiers with the diagnosis of 'effort syndrome'. Results vary from the excessively optimistic claim by Eysenck (1952) that 'two thirds of a group of neurotic patients will recover or improve to a marked extent within about two years of the onset of their illness, whether they are treated by means of psychotherapy or not', to the much more cautious comment by Malan *et al.* (1975) that the rate for those who improve dynamically is nearer 25%. Follow-up studies have varied very much in their results for outcome, and the reasons for this have been the differences between the samples of patients assessed, widely different methods of assessment carried out, and various errors in these methods. Errors in forming the sample studied have been quite common; an inadequate number of patients followed-up will prevent any conclusions being drawn about differences within the sample; the sample technique may have been faulty, for example, a study which claimed to be of 'neurosis' but was carried out on hospital in-patients who had to pay to be there. A study compared two different types of treatment for neurosis, claiming much better results for one form of treatment than the other. The patients had in fact been allowed to choose which type of treatment they would prefer, and those who were more 'psychologically minded' were more likely to choose one type of treatment and also had a better prognosis.

One hundred patients, considered to be suffering from neurotic disorders when attending their family doctors, were followed-up after one year (Mann *et al.*, 1981). The severity of psychiatric morbidity and the quality of social life were found to be the factors which predicted psychiatric state at the end of the year. These authors considered that symptoms, personality and social state could be considered independently in terms of prognosis. Continuous psychiatric morbidity throughout the year of study was found in patients who were older, more likely to show abnormality and to have received a diagnosis of depression.

Neurotic patients were compared with a matched non-neurotic sample (Sims and Gooding, 1975). Patients who were previously treated in hospital for neurosis were compared for outcome with a group, matched for age and sex, of people who had received surgery for varicose veins in the same year. A similar method of follow-up was used for the previous neurotic and varicose vein patients, and a global assessment of outcome was carried out taking into account symptoms, requirements for treatment over the years, alcohol and drug dependence, and also the extent of social disruption including problems in the areas of work, home relationships, marital and sexual relationship and material management. At follow-up 90% of the surgical group were found to have a satisfactory outcome on this measure of neurotic disability whilst only 44% of the previous neurotic group had done as well. Only 1 in 10 'normal' people showed more than minimal symptoms of social disturbance resulting from neurosis, but more than half of those originally considered severely neurotic remained conspicuously disadvantaged. The difference between the two groups was highly significant, and is shown in figure 5.1. The General Health Questionnaire (described later) also discriminated between the two groups with a substantial majority of the previous neurotics achieving high, and hence pathological, scores. Only 40% of the neurotic group were considered to have normal personalities at follow-up; this was similar to the proportion of these patients found at initial admission to hospital 12 years before. Using the same criteria for assessing personality, 75% of the 'normal' surgical group was found to have a normal personality.

For the prediction of outcome in 'minor psychiatric disorders' (neuroses), social circumstances are probably the most important factors according to Huxley *et al.* (1979) who followed-up 52 patients at one year. They investigated such circumstances as dissatis-

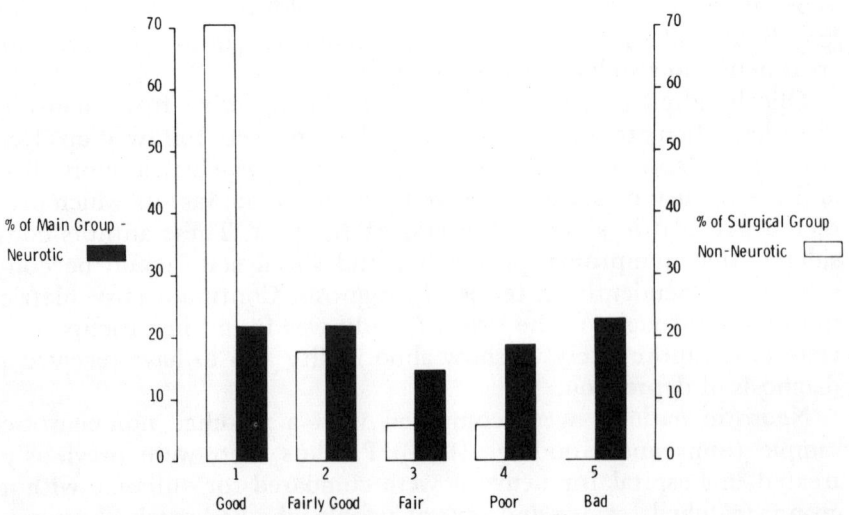

Figure 5.1   Total outcome at follow-up: Neurotic group compared with surgical group

faction with social contacts and leisure activities, housing and social class, as well as symptomatic and constitutional variables.

Other studies have also shown that neurosis is not a benign condition. Niskanen *et al.* (1974) reckoned that two thirds of neurotic inpatients had an unsatisfactory outcome at follow-up, with either a chronic course incapacitating the patient, or the occurrence of psychosis.

Dependence upon Drugs, Alcohol, Tobacco and People

A single man, aged 28, was treated for anxiety and phobic symptoms. He had great difficulty with mixing, feeling tongue-tied and inferior to the people he met. He worked in a steel foundry, and recently he had been walking the three miles home from work, because he had experienced a panic attack on the bus. During treatment his anxiety symptoms diminished with sedative drugs, but he did not allow himself to become involved in group therapy. At follow-up 12 years later, he was living on his own under poor conditions in a flat in a large old house. He was unemployed and was drinking about 10 pints of beer each night. He had no friends apart from the people he met in the pub. He said that he could not sleep unless he 'had a drink'. He had served two prison sentences for theft, obtaining money for drink.

It could be anticipated that severely neurotic people are more likely than others to become dependent upon alcohol and drugs, because the problems they experience are particularly those that provoke heavy drinking or drug dependence, and such people are more likely to respond to treatment by becoming dependent upon it. They experience more problems than other people, and amongst neurotics there is a higher proportion of personalities prone to addiction.

In fact at 12-year follow-up, over 10% of previous neurotic patients showed established dependence on either alcohol or drugs with withdrawal symptoms present, problems arising from excessive consumption of the drug or alcohol, or overdosage (Sims, 1975a). Interestingly, at follow-up 23% of these previous neurotic patients were total abstainers from alcohol; this is almost twice the rate expected for a population of this age and sex composition; half the sample took no regular psychotropic medication at all.

Those dependent on alcohol or drugs had a much worse outcome at follow-up than the rest of previously treated neurotic patients. More unexpectedly, those who had developed dependence by the time of follow-up had showed a more severe degree of neurosis at the time they were treated in hospital, and were more likely to have been deemed disordered in personality. This was before they had developed their problem with abuse of drugs or alcohol. It seems therefore, that more severely neurotic patients are at greater risk from developing dependence. Alcohol and drug dependence was much commoner amongst those previously treated for neurosis, but not then dependent, than in the general adult population.

Smokers are particularly likely to light up when they are anxious or stressed. One might expect that a neurotic population is likely to have a higher proportion of smokers, and that those who smoke are likely to smoke more than non-neurotic smokers. From a survey of smoking habits before admission in a group of patients treated in hospital for neurosis compared with a surgical control group and with general population surveys, the neurotics were more likely to be smokers; those who smoked burned considerably more cigarettes per day; they tended to start smoking at a younger age and they were more likely to inhale deeply (Salmons and Sims, 1981).

Neurotic patients are more emotionally dependent upon other people than those without neurosis, and they make more demands upon other people. For example, a sample of patients with a diagnosis of neurosis made heavy demands upon their general practitioners, with frequent attendance at surgery, multiple complaints, a large variety of symptomatic treatments prescribed and frequent referral to hospital specialists. This was quantified by comparing the weight of general practitioner case files for a sample of neurotic patients compared with age and sex matched non-neurotic patients from the same practices. The neurotic files were found to be very much heavier. It is quite clear that such neurotic patients also have more physical illnesses than others.

In the Harlow study (Taylor and Chave, 1964), it was found that those patients showing subclinical neurosis syndrome made more demands on their family doctors and upon hospital services for treatment of physical and psychological symptoms; they made more complaint of symptoms and they had more illnesses. Various studies in general practice have confirmed the increased demands for treatment; there is also an increase in other illnesses amongst neurotic patients.

Neurosis to Psychosis

Does neurotic decompensation occur, with the patient eventually deteriorating into psychosis? Some psychiatric theories have seen neurosis and psychosis as a diagnostic continuum, with so called 'borderline states' merging the neuroses on one side with psychoses on the other. In such a scheme, neurosis is seen as an adaptive reaction for coping with unacceptable unpleasant emotion, but there is a limit to the degree of adaptation that is possible and, if this be exceeded, the integrity of the person is shattered, reality judgment is lost and overt psychosis supersedes. If this were so, if neurosis were a 'form fruste' of psychosis, then at follow-up of severe neuroses over a long time one would expect a considerable shift towards psychosis.

In 14 follow-up studies of neurosis which cite a rate for the subsequent development of psychosis, the figure for change from neurosis to psychosis varied from 0% to 13.8%, with a mean of 5.8%. In my follow-up, 117 neurotic patients who were treated in hospital were interviewed; three of these patients at 12 year follow-up were diagnosed as affective psychosis, and two as schizophrenia (Sims, 1976). Thus five patients (4%) had become psychotic in 12 years. None of the three with affective psychosis had shown a manic phase, but they had required electronconvulsive therapy for depression subsequent to the admission during which they were deemed neurotic. The case notes at the initial treatment of the two patients subsequently schizophrenic both showed a query for the presence of schizophrenia. As in other studies, an extremely low shift from severe neurosis to psychosis was found, more compatible with misdiagnosis than true progression from neurosis to psychosis.

Mortality

An important, even sinister, finding from follow-up studies in neurosis is the fact that there is an increased mortality. Brown (1965) described an increased risk for neurotics to suffer from physical illness, and that illness was more likely to become chronic.

It was also found in a rural community in Spain that neurosis and physical illness were likely to coexist in the same patients (Vázquez Barquero *et al.*, 1981). Of those showing neurotic manifestations, 42% of males and 39% of females also showed physical pathology.

Neurosis is well recognised to be a prolonged and irritating condition, but it is very rarely invoked as a cause of death. Mortality Statistics for England and Wales record only 564 deaths with a diagnosis of neuroses and related disorders (International Classification of Diseases, 300-309) for the year 1979 (OPCS, 1980). Of these 503 were for alcoholism and drug dependence, 23 for anorexia nervosa and only 13 claimed for neurotic disorders (ICD 300). Neurosis disturbs no vital function and is not, in itself, ever lethal. However neurotics tend to die prematurely. Mortality studies in neurosis have looked at different samples of patients. Babigian and Odoroff (1969) studied the mortality of patients from the Monroe County Case

Register in U.S.A. They found the observed mortality for neurotic patients to be about twice the expected rate for the general population. Keehn *et al.* (1974) followed up U.S. Army veterans who had been medically discharged from the service for psychoneurosis 20 years before. They found the relative risk of mortality to be 1.4 times the rate of a control group of subjects in a Life Insurance scheme matched for age, sex, race and service features.

We followed up 1482 patients with a diagnosis of neurosis 11 years after hospital treatment (Sims and Prior, 1978). Ninety one per cent of patients were traced. One hundred and thirty nine patients had died, and this was a highly significant increase in mortality compared with expectation. Relative risk of death (which is the ratio of observed mortality to expected mortality for a sample) for these neurotic patients was 1.7. There was, as expected, a marked increase of deaths from suicide and accident, but there was also a highly significant increase from natural causes (relative risk 1.6), as shown in table 5.1 which summarises data for the 1482 neurotic patients.

Suicide and accidents did not particularly concentrate amongst those whose previous diagnosis was depressive neurosis. It could be shown that for almost all those whom coroners decide were accidental deaths or open verdicts, their mental state or psychiatric

Table 5.1   *Observed and Expected Mortality in 1482 neurotic subjects at follow-up*

	Deaths — expected number	Deaths— observed number	Probability	Relative risk
All causes of death	83.92	139	< 0.001	1.7
Diseases of the nervous, respiratory and circulatory systems	46.64	75	< 0.001	1.6
Self-inflicted death	2.07	14	< 0.001	6.8
Accidents, poisoning and violence, excluding self-inflicted death	3.69	17	< 0.001	4.6
Remainder	31.52	33	—	1.0

condition had contributed, at least in part, to their death ('quasi-suicide'). A previous diagnosis of 'hysteria' (most often hysterical personality disorder) was particularly associated with quasisuicide.

An example of quasisuicide would be a man who was killed by a railway train 5 years after treatment for neurotic depressive symptoms. At the inquest (as noted by the Coroner) the engine driver said that he had seen the man beside the tracks, had put on his brakes, but at the last moment the man had stepped in front of the engine rather than get out of the way. The legal verdict was accidental death as it was thought that perhaps the man was trying to avoid the train, had become confused and jumped the wrong way. The psychiatric assessment was quasisuicide, as he had expressed suicidal ideas whilst an in-patient initially; he had taken an overdose two years before his death; it certainly appeared that his mental state had contributed to his death.

Amongst deaths from natural causes, cardiovascular, neurological and respiratory deaths were significantly increased. There was no increase above expectation for deaths from cancer. Arteriosclerosis appeared to be the major pathological process accounting for excess mortality and this raises questions of constitutional factors, neurotic symptoms as produced in arteriosclerosis and the possible role of smoking (Sims and Prior, 1982). We have no information on blood lipids and blood pressure recordings in neurotic patients without physical illness.

When the case histories of neurotic patients who subsequently died were compared with those who were still alive at follow-up, it was

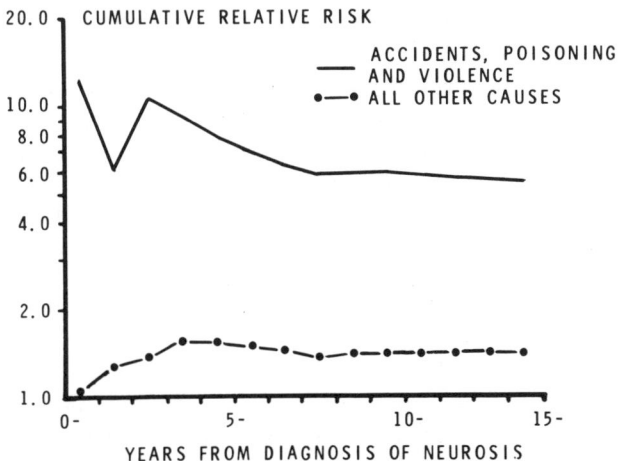

Figure 5.2   Mortality in severe neurosis

found that those who died had shown a more severe degree of neurosis initially (Sims and Rudge, 1979). It is likely that this increased death risk is a feature of neurosis itself, and not of misdiagnosis at the time of treatment. Initially following treatment, the relative risk for death amongst neurotic patients from natural causes is not increased; it only reaches a high rate after about 3-4 years (figure 5.2). Conversely the greatest risk of death from suicide and accident is in the year or two immediately after treatment, suggesting that some arrangements to maintain contact with the patient would be justified for longer than is at present usual.

Mortality increased above expectation is revealed when previously treated neurotic patients are followed-up. This increase is not only from suicide and accidents but also from natural causes. The mortality rate is higher with more severe neurosis. Is premature death more likely following the breaking of 'affectional bonds'? The evidence does not yet support or contradict this notion.

Evaluaton of Severity and Outcome of Neurosis

The Need for Assessment

The point has been made earlier that everyone is neurotic at least to some extent. However there is a great variation in the degree of neurosis, that is in the disabling quality of symptoms and the destructiveness of their effect on social behaviour. In order to ascertain the degree of this disability, it is necessary to measure it. There has been increasing interest over the last few years in assessment of the efficacy of treatment, especially of the various psychotherapies.

The neurotic patient either fails to cope adequately with his life circumstances, or alternatively copes but with considerable difficulty. To decide if treatment is effective, it is necessary to be able to measure relevant features about the person before and after treatment using a valid, reliable, quantitative method. This is the only way we can get away from vague over-optimistic claims being made for all sorts of different treatments. The various areas of importance in terms of disability from neurosis can be summarised into two main realms (table 5.2). First, is the symptomatic state which assesses the presence and severity of symptoms, and their direct effects on life course; for example, death, wholly or partly attributed to the mental state; requirements of hospitalisation; medication taken, and so on. The second is the social state; this encompasses disruption relating to work, marital and sexual state, family and home relationships and material management. For measurement of the social state these dif-

Table 5.2   Total outcome in neurosis

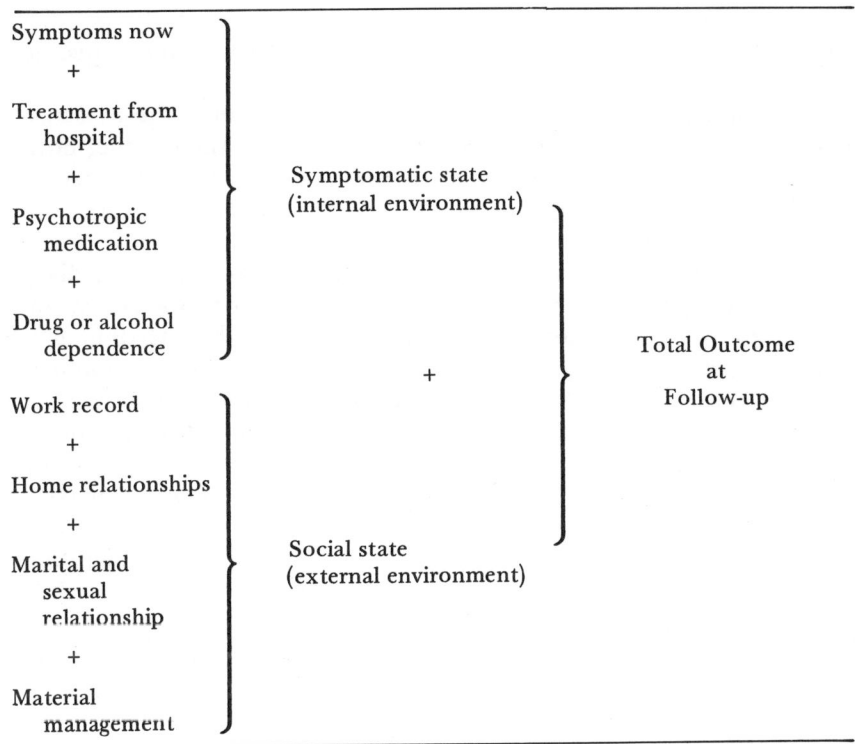

ferent areas require to be evaluated separately, and then summed to give a composite score.

The differences in the presentation and severity of neurotic symptoms between different populations is very important. For any research study, careful selection of the sample is vital. This is probably the stage at which more psychiatric research is rendered invalid than any other. Conclusions drawn from the findings of one sample cannot necessarily be applied to any other sample; it has first to be demonstrated that the two populations have similar characteristics.

Instruments for Evaluating Neurosis

The neurotic characteristics of individuals in a group have been assessed in many different ways. A straight forward counting of heads is the simplest, although this has potential pitfalls. As an example of simple counting in a follow-up study, one method used to assess outcome following self-poisoning is to record the number of repeat overdoses in a defined time in each of two groups of people treated in a different way.

Questionnaires have frequently been used to assess the presence of symptoms; these have considerable problems in their usage, both in the subject understanding what is asked, and in the relevance of the data collected (Oppenheim, 1966). Postal questionnaires are unlikely to produce a high enough response rate in previous neurotic patients; one cannot ask complicated questions, nor subsidiary questions needing further explanation; one cannot probe for meaning, and one does not know who actually completed the questionnaire. When used, a questionnaire should be so designed that the respondent can answer without irritation. The questions must be relevant, easily comprehended, and give a response that can be coded by the interviewer. Because questions are so easily misunderstood, their wording is very important, and for this reason a pilot study is always needed to find out how subjects will respond. Questions must be specific and asked in simple language avoiding vague words and ambiguities. Questions which lead the subject or presume a certain answer ('When did you last smoke cannabis?') must be avoided. Hypothetical questions and those that embarrass the respondent are not likely to be answered satisfactorily.

Check lists may be used for assessing symptomatic or social state in neurosis. For example, economic state has been investigated asking the subject what items they own from a list of household goods (refrigerator, telephone, lawn-mower, etc.). Rating scales, which are a sophistication of check lists in that individual items are weighted are very liable to error, especially from the halo effect of a rating on one item being carried over to another item, but self-rating scales have been used to learn about the patient's own emotions, for example, the Leeds Self Assessment Scale (Snaith *et al.*, 1976), part of which is demonstrated in table 5.3. With visual analogue scales, the subject makes a mark to record his present state, on a straight line (10 cm) the ends of which represent two extremes of a quality. For example, the patient could be asked to mark on the line his present mood when one end had the statement, 'I feel miserable', and the other end, 'I feel fine', as in figure 5.3. Explanation to the patient is very important to ensure that he understands what he is supposed to be doing.

Inventories are a refinement on check lists in which the respondent completes the questionnaire in such a way as to provide a profile of his state. The General Health Questionnaire, part of which is shown

Table 5.3   *Self-rating: Part of the Leeds Self Assessment Scale*

Please indicate how you are feeling now, or how you have been feeling in the last day or two, by <u>UNDERLINING</u> the correct response to each of the following items:

---

4. I feel anxious when I go out of the house on my own	a)	<u>Yes definitely</u>
	b)	Yes sometimes
	c)	No not much
	d)	No not at all
5. I have lost interest in things	a)	Yes definitely
	b)	<u>Yes sometimes</u>
	c)	No not much
	d)	No not at all
6. I get palpitations or a sensation of "butterflies" in my stomach or chest	a)	Yes definitely
	b)	<u>Yes sometimes</u>
	c)	No not much
	d)	No not at all
7. I still enjoy the things I used to do	a)	Yes definitely
	b)	Yes sometimes
	c)	No not much
	d)	<u>No not at all</u>

---

in table 5.4, is an example of an inventory that has been widely used in surveys of different populations looking for the presence of psychiatric morbidity (Goldberg and Blackwell, 1970). It is, for example, used to decide what proportion of a population in general practice is suffering from emotional symptoms. The Minnesota Multiphasic Personality Inventory (MMPI) and its modifications have been used extensively for investigating destructive patterns of personality and behaviour.

Grids are two-dimensional inventories. For assessing aspects of neurotic disorder, the Repertory Grid has been extensively used to examine the inner world of the neurotic person, his 'semantic space',

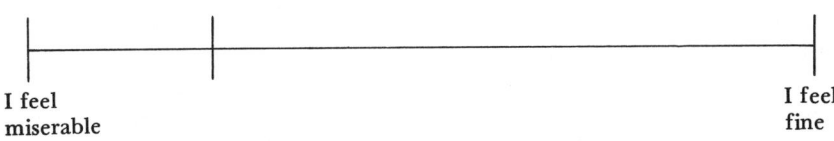

I feel
miserable

I feel
fine

Figure 5.3   A visual analogue scale for mood

Table 5.4   General Health Questionnaire: A part

We should like to know if you have had any medical complaints, and how your health has been in general, <u>over the past few weeks.</u> Please answer ALL the questions on the following pages simply by underlining the answer which you think most nearly applies to you. Remember that we want to know about present and recent complaints, not those that you had in the past.

It is important that you try to answer ALL the questions.

Thank you very much for your co-operation.

HAVE YOU RECENTLY:

34. –	kept feeling afraid to say anything to people in case you made a fool of yourself?	Not at all	No more than usual	<u>Rather more than usual</u>	Much more than usual
35. –	felt that you are playing a useful part in things?	More so than usual	Same as usual	Less useful than usual	<u>Much less useful</u>
36. –	felt capable of making decisions about things?	More so than usual	Same as usual	Less so than usual	<u>Much less capable</u>
37. –	felt you're just not able to make a start on anything?	Not at all	<u>No more than usual</u>	Rather more than usual	Much more than usual
38. –	felt yourself dreading everything that you have to do?	Not at all	No more than usual	<u>Rather more than usual</u>	Much more than usual

how he evaluates different parts of his environment (Ryle, 1975). For example, it can give a two-dimensional picture of the way a person sees himself, and how he would like himself to be compared with other people important to him. A girl, aged 20 had taken four overdoses in the last two years, and had slashed her wrists ten times during that time. She had not been to her work in an insurance office for nearly three years. She felt herself to be a complete failure. She described the significant people in her life, and from these descriptions a repertory grid was constructed. How she saw the 'elements', in this case those people in her life who mattered in relation to the 'constructs' (the description of these people) is represented in figure

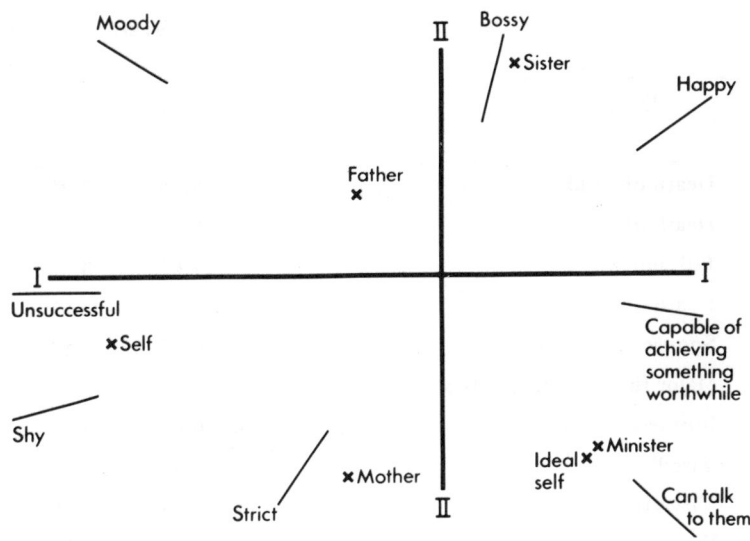

Figure 5.4   Repertory grid: simplified form for a patient

5.4, which shows the first two principal components after computing her quantified assessment of each element for each construct.

She considers herself to be extremely 'unsuccessful' and 'shy', very different from everyone else, and especially different from how she would like to be (her ideal self). She considered her sister to be both 'bossy' and 'happy', her father to be 'moody' and her mother 'strict'. She wanted to be like her minister, whom she did not know well but idealised, as 'a person one can talk to' and 'capable of achieving something worthwhile'. The constructs are vectors or directions and 'happy' was exactly opposed to herself; that is, she was very unhappy. The elements and the wording of the constructs were chosen by her; the repertory grid is therefore a map of her semantic space, the way she sees her world and the people in it.

An index sums the answers to different questions to give a score. For example, the Middlesex Hospital Questionnaire gives scores for different neurotic syndromes, such as obsessionality (Crown and Crisp, 1966). Psychiatric diagnosis has been standardised for research purposes using the Present State Examination (Wing *et al.*, 1974). This does not use neurosis as a diagnostic category, but neuroses are represented separately (tension, lack of energy, etc.).

There have been interesting developments from sociological theory to construct instruments for measuring social network, that is the quality and quantity of human relationships of the subject. An example of such an instrument is the Interviewer Schedule for Social

Table 5.5   *Mean scores for perceptions of life events (after Paykel et al., (1971))*

Rank order	Event	Mean	SC
1	Death of child	19.33	2.22
2	Death of spouse	18.76	3.21
3	Jail sentence	17.60	3.56
4	Death of family member	17.21	3.69
5	Spouse unfaithful	16.78	4.14
6	Major financial difficulties	16.57	3.83
7	Business failure	16.46	3.71
8	'Fired'	16.45	4.20
9	Miscarriage or stillbirth	16.34	4.59
10	Divorce	16.18	4.95
	+	+	+
52	Marriage	5.61	5.67
53	Promotion	5.39	4.90
54	Minor personal illness	5.20	4.29
55	Move in same city	5.14	4.49
56	Birth of child (father) or adoption	5.13	5.45
57	Begin education	5.09	4.48
58	Child becomes engaged	4.53	4.57
59	Become engaged	3.70	4.64
60	Wanted pregnancy	3.56	5.39
61	Child married (approved)	2.94	3.75

Interaction (ISSI) which investigates the personal network, both close affectional bonds and more diffuse relationships (Henderson *et al.*, 1980). A scale has been constructed by Paykel *et al.* (1971) of life events. 373 people including patients and their relatives were asked to make judgments on a 0 to 20 equal interval rating scale as to how upsetting each of 61 events in a list was considered to be. The most and the least upsetting items from this list are shown in table 5.5. These scales and schedules, inventories and grids described in this section are only a small sample of the numerous tests that have been used to evaluate different aspects of neurosis.

Tracing

In order to measure outcome, previously assessed patients must be followed-up. A vital step in this medical follow-up procedure is finding the patients-tracing. Many follow-up studies of neurosis have been satisfied with a low tracing rate, for example less than 60% of the original treatment group were found in seven out of 40 follow-up studies of neurosis. Sixty per cent tracing is generally easy to achieve but higher rates are considerably more difficult. However, it was demonstrated for neurotics that findings are not uniform for the whole sample traced (Sims, 1973). For example, although there were only three deaths found amongst the first 59% of patients traced at follow-up, a further 18 deaths were discovered in the subsequent 38% of previous patients traced. In this study 186 past patients were followed-up with 97% tracing.

A higher tracing rate is obtained by home visits than other methods. Postal surveys will often obtain about 40–50% response rate, although response has varied in different studies from 10% to 90% according to motivation of the respondents. Follow-up in which the previous patient is asked to return to the hospital out-patient department will often achieve about 60% response. It is always important to decide whether a high tracing rate is necessary or not before planning the method of follow-up.

Interviewing at Follow-up

Information about the patient may be given by the patient himself, relatives or friends, the therapist or a researcher working independently from the therapist. If accounts from these four people; the patient, his relative, the therapist and the independent interviewer, were obtained, and they were all to agree, then three of the accounts would have been redundant. However, if they disagree one is left with the problem of whose story to accept. This is a recurring problem in the interpretation of interviews. Another important consideration is where should the interview take place. It is often convenient to bring the patient for a research interview to the interviewer, for example at hospital, but a higher tracing rate may be achieved by interviewing at home, and the information given by the patient when relaxed in his own home may be of greater validity, although the interviewer has to learn how to combat the television and the friendly Golden Labrador!

It is difficult at first interview to distinguish the effects of the present condition from the person's underlying premorbid personality. There are a number of practical problems in the ascertainment of information from the patient, both how to collect the information and what it means. Is the information reliable?; that is, will you get the same answer next time?; and valid, that is, does it really answer the questions that needed to be clarified? Can the account of the patient's symptoms be made quantitative? The format of the interview will be determined by the answers to these questions. It will be necessary to start this type of research with a pilot study to determine whether the interview should be structured, semi-structured or informal.

Attention needs to be given to the actual process of obtaining the interview, of gaining access to the subject of enquiry. How questions are asked, the precise wording, matters a great deal for the validity of response. How the answers are recorded will affect the eventual quality of information obtained. When assessing the patient's history the sequence of events occurring during his life is important.

Studying the Process of Change

In the same way that the onset of neurosis may be related to the presence of adverse circumstances (life events), its improvement is associated with significant factors in the environment (neutralising life events). Frequently when a patient gets better he is able to give some account of the reasons for this improvement, and he may be correct or misguided in his conclusions. It is of very considerable interest to find out how these changes occur; and, particularly with reference to planning treatment, it is very important to evaluate the processes (Malan, 1976; Garfield and Bergin, 1978; Sifneos, 1979; Crown, 1980).

What is treatment, to be effective, trying to achieve? There can be three levels of intention in treatment for neurosis. First, the aim may be the relief of symptoms; this may or may not be associated with improved adjustment in other areas of life. Second, one is looking for long term changes with fewer symptoms and better social adjustment and ways of coping. Third is to give the patient or client a satisfying experience; this may or may not have any long term consequences. Psychotherapy and related treatments are expensive, very demanding in the time and skill of therapists, and stressful to both patient and therapist. Most doctors and their patients would, therefore, consider that the most worthwhile endeavour is to attempt the second objective, that is, a long term improvement in many areas of life.

In assessment of the efficacy of treatment methods in neurosis there are three variables to consider. The therapist, the patient and the social situation in which they interact. A great deal of attention has been given to the qualities of the therapist (Parloff *et al.*, 1978).

The beneficial qualities of the therapist have been described in terms of accurate empathy, non-possessive warmth and genuineness (Truax and Carkhuff, 1967). These variables are extremely difficult to measure and later studies have not always validated the earlier findings. The processes that take place in therapy have been investigated to assess which are important for improvement of the patient (Strupp and Hadley, 1979).

It is not only improvement that may occur in psychotherapy, deterioration occurs in a certain proportion of patients (Strupp *et al.*, 1978). Certain characteristics of the leader in group psychotherapy have a deleterious effect upon the members of the group, such as 'high stimulus input, aggressivity, charisma, support, intrusiveness and individual (as opposed to interpersonal or group) forms. The most vulnerable subjects were those with low self-concept and unrealistically large expectations and anticipations of change' (Yalom and Lieberman, 1971).

The social situation encompassing patient and therapist includes both the methods of treatment and the setting in which it occurs. Sloane and others (1975) have made a careful comparison between the effectiveness of dynamic psychotherapy and behavioural psychotherapy. In practice both methods were found to be effective, and the differences between the two did not seem to be based upon theoretical considerations. For a variety of reasons there have been very few studies comparing different methods of treatment but this is clearly an area which requires considerably more work in future.

Measuring Outcome

Follow-up studies are essential for the assessment of efficacy of treatment and also for studying the natural history of neurosis. There are three stages in such studies; first is the assessment of the initial status of patients; second, after a time-interval, carrying out the follow-up process with tracing the members of the cohort; and third is measurement of outcome. Forming the initial sample has already been discussed, for meaningful results at a later stage this must be done well.

One of the important processes for a trial of treatment is the comparison of two groups of patients, one with the form of treatment under investigation, and the other (control group) receiving another form of treatment, preferably one for which the results of treatment are known. This methodology has been worked out for drug trials where double-blind cross-over has become the model for evaluation of new treatment (Doll, 1959). Patients are randomly allocated to one of two groups. In one group the patients start with the new method of treatment which is to be assessed, and at the half way stage are changed to the known form of treatment. In the other group the patients receive treatment in the reverse order. Neither doctor nor patient knows which order of treatment any individual patient is receiving. Assessments are carried out before treatment, at the time of cross-over and at the end of the trial.

Unfortunately this simple model for trial of treatment has not proved possible for psychotherapy for a number of reasons. It has not been possible to form adequate control groups of patients receiving other forms of treatment, or no treatment at all. It has not proved practicable to allocate patients randomly to a treatment and a non-treatment group. Finding methods of assessment has also been difficult. One account of an attempt at such a treatment trial for psychotherapy in fact ended as a description of the problems that prevented the trial being completed (Candy *et al.*, 1972). A possible way of avoiding some of these difficulties would be to compare patients in two different settings by assessing their likely prognosis in terms of the presence of factors predictive of poor outcome (Sims, 1982). If it could be shown that the expected outcome of the two groups was approximately equal and subsequent follow-up showed marked differences between them, one factor to explain this could be the differences in treatment.

Assessment of the status of patients should be carried out at the beginning and end of treatment. Data such as age, sex, marital status and social class are obviously of importance, so also is the clinical description of the patients in terms of their presenting symptoms, duration of illness, age at which symptoms occurred, clinical diagnosis, and so on. It is very important to assess patients fully in all areas of their social life; that is in those areas listed above of work, marital and sexual status, home and family matters and material management. Various personality assessments and enquiries concerning personal health will also be relevant. Finally, information regarding particular characteristics of the sample, for example, if they were all phobic, the natures and detailed descriptions of their phobias, will be ascertained. Information known about neurotic patients at the time of treatment is potentially predictive of outcome, and it is important to have assessed these areas.

There is no single measure which gives an accurate evaluation of patients outcome, and so it is necessary to construct a scale or index that incorporates different assessments; including symptomatic and social state detailed above. It is important how one takes into consideration those patients who are lost at follow-up, both those who have not been traced and will have to be excluded, and those who have died. If their death has been associated with their mental state, they should be included under 'very poor' outcome. Successful tracing, but refused interview is also an important category that must be considered. Follow-up studies in neurosis are vital in obtaining information and in working towards the assessment of efficacy of treatment, but they present many practical difficulties.

The Neurotic Paradigm

The factors that predict poor outcome in neurosis are not independent or isolated, but interdependent. Thus abnormality of personality is associated with a cluster of factors which affect prognosis adversely. Problems in relationships in one area of life will result in difficulties in other areas, because the patient is still the same awkward person mixing with others who have in common with him their human frailties. If a patient copes poorly in one part of his life, he is likely to do so in other parts as well, because he has the same attitude and problems with relationships arising from his behaviour.

Many follow-up studies in neurosis have found items of information known about the patient at the time of treatment to be predictive of outcome. Some factors, such as diagnosis and nature of symptoms, social disruption, premorbid personality, duration of symptoms and precipitating factors recur regularly and are probably of general predictive relevance. Other factors which are specific to individual studies probably reflect the characteristics of that particular patient sample. The factors mentioned and the number of papers in which that factor is mentioned in 32 studies are summarised in figure 5.5.

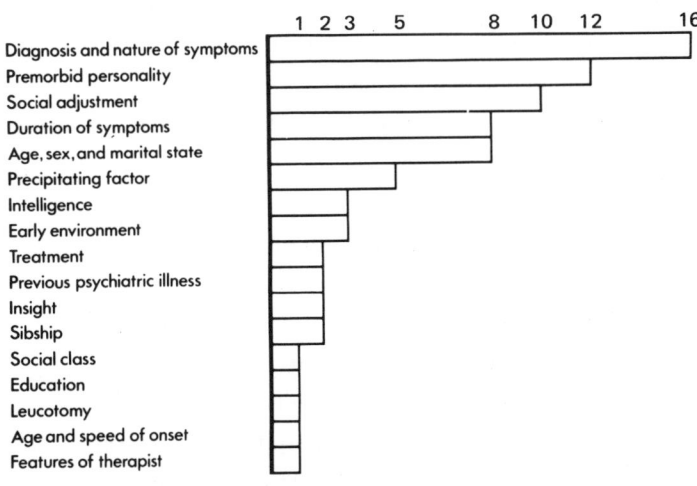

Figure 5.5   Factors mentioned as predictive in follow-up studies of neurosis

In a follow-up study of 146 neurotic patients treated in hospital at 12 year follow-up, 79 factors were investigated to see whether they predicted prognosis (Sims, 1975b). Twenty six factors were found to be significantly predictive of poor outcome and these are listed in table 5.6.

In other chapters it has been stressed to what extent neurosis is a

Table 5.6   Factors predictive of poor outcome in neurosis

1. Precipitation of illness described by patient to sexual, marital, family or occupational problem

2. Length of present illness more than 6 years

3. Age under 20 at development of present illness

4. Primary diagnosis of personality disorder

5. Abnormal personality

6. Absence of social symptoms in neurotic illness

7. Unemployment for more than 3 months before inception

8. Frequent change of employment

9. Work record conspicuously unsatisfactory

10. Unsatisfactory relationship with spouse or cohabitee

11. Conspicuous behaviour or personality problem of spouse or cohabitee

12. Age of spouse at time of marriage less than 20, or more than 25

13. Presence of criminal record

14. Problems with accommodation or financial state

15. Social help required during treatment

16. Disturbed relationships between parents during patient's childhood

17. Unhappy childhood

18. Considered unsuitable for psychotherapy

19. Received further treatment since inception

20. Admission as in-patient rather than day-patient or out-patient

21. Course during treatment recorded as 'worse' or 'unchanged'

22. State on discharge 'worse' or 'unchanged'

23. Non-attendance at follow-up appointments

24. Large number of letters written from hospital about patient

25. Large number of pages of case notes written about patient

26. Prognosis at time of discharge considered 'poor'

process rather than a single event. There is a degree of inevitability which dictates that neurotic thinking will be followed by a neurotic pattern of behaviour; and the sense of failure that this behaviour engenders causes a further sequence of neurotic thinking that in its turn precipitates further neurotic behaviour. This may explain how the neurotic predictors become interdependent. This is represented in the 'Neurotic Paradigm', in figure 5.6.

Personality problems and, in the patient's own description, an unhappy childhood are the seedbed for the growth of further difficulties; such an unsatisfactory background places the individual in a worse social situation from which to cope with the problems and crises of life. Trying to cope from this position of disadvantage limits his available future choices. His personality difficulties make it intrisically more likely that there will be further problems with relationships, such as at work and in marriage. Similarly, because of this neurotic disposition, he is a less attractive person to take into employment or to choose as a husband; for this reason his occupational and marital choices are limited to a smaller number of possibilities, which may be less congenial and more likely to result in subsequent problems. Through having contracted an unsatisfactory marriage or obtained an unsuitable job, further problems are likely to result in the areas of work, marriage and the general management of life situations.

People with neurosis are likely to describe the difficulties caused by internal conflicts in terms of their social repercussions; it is usually that 'other people don't treat me properly', rather than recognising that the problem in relationships arises from inside himself as a person. He has got himself into a situation in life in which it

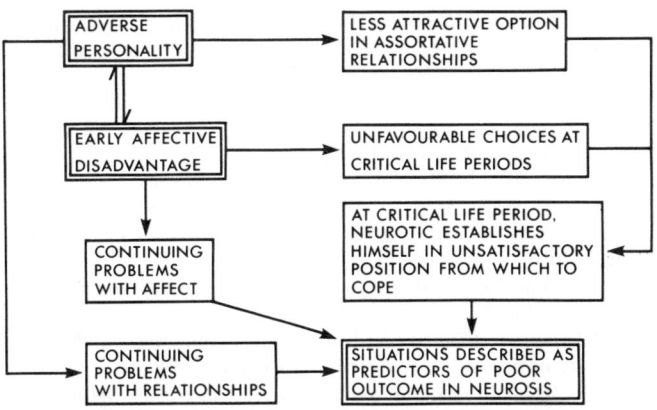

Figure 5.6   A neurotic paradigm: 'one forever out of his element'

would be more difficult for anyone to cope because of the multitude of difficulties that have arisen, and also he is a person who because of his self-doubt intrinsically finds it more difficult to cope with the ordinary problems of everyday life.

The neurotic patient's early affective disadvantage, described by him as 'having had an unhappy childhood', or 'a lot of rows at home' in his original family, is likely to show itself in continuing problems with mood; the unhappy child may inexorably develop into the unhappy adult. The problem in his personality development will not only have caused difficulties in 'assortative relationships' at the time of making major life decisions, it will also continue to cause problems with relationships in the present.

The difficulty, for various reasons, that the neurotic patient has in coping, his continuing problems with feelings, and his continuing problems with relationships are likely to result in further situations which could be described as predictors of poor outcome in neurosis. These in their turn promote the continuation of neurotic symptoms. It is because there is such a concerted assault from so many directions, and in such a consistently destructive way that the justification of the term 'illness' for neurosis becomes appropriate. It is, also, this synergistic effect of a multitude of adverse factors that creates the difficulty of treatment in neurosis. Any effective treatment will have to try and act at several different points in the paradigm at the same time to reverse the feeling of inevitability that is engendered.

Bibliography

Babigian, H.M. and Odoroff, C.L. (1969). The mortality experience of a population with psychiatric illness. *Am. J. Psychiat.*, 126, 4, 470–480.

Bronte, Charlotte (1848). *Shirley*

Brown, A.C. (1965). *The General Morbidity of Neurotic Patients*, Cambridge, M.D. Thesis

Candy, J., Alpha, S.H.G., Cawley, R.H., Hilderbrand, H.P., Malan, D.H., Marks, I.M. and Wilson, J. (1972). A feasibility study for a control trial of formal psychotherapy. *Psychol. Med.*, 2, 345–362

Cooper, B. and Morgan, H.G. (1973). *Epidemiological Psychiatry*, Thomas, Springfield, Illinois

Crown, S. (1980). The future of the psychotherapies. In: *Priorities in Psychiatric Research* (Ed. Lader, M.), Wiley, Chichester

Crown, S. and Crisp, A. (1966). A short clinical diagnostic self-rating scale for psychoneurotic patients. *Br. J. Psychiat.*, 112, 917–923

Doll, R. (1959). *Medical Surveys and Clinical Trials* (Ed. Witts, L.J.), Oxford University Press, London

Eysenck, H.J. (1952). The effects of psychotherapy: An evaluation. *J. Consult. Psychol.*, 16, 319–324

Garfield, S.L. and Bergin, A.E. (Eds) (1978). *Handbook of Psychotherapy and Behaviour Change: An Empirical Analysis*, 2nd edn, John Wiley, New York

Goldberg, D.P. and Blackwell, B. (1970). Psychiatric illness in general practice. A detailed study using a new method of case identification. *Br. med. J.*, 2, 439–443

Grant, R.T. (1925). Observation on the after histories of men suffering from the effort syndrome. *Heart*, 12, 121–142

Greer, H.S. and Cawley, R.H. (1966). *Some Observations on the Natural History of Neurotic Illness*, Australasian Medical Publishing Co. Ltd., Sydney

Hare, E.H. and Wing, J.K. (1970). *Psychiatric Epidemiology*, OUP, London

Henderson, S., Duncan-Jones, P., Byrne, D.G. and Scott, R. (1980). Measuring social relationships: the Interview Schedule for Social Interaction. *Psychol. Med.*, 10, 723–734

Huxley, P.J., Goldberg, D.P., Maguire, G.P. and Kinley, V.A. (1979). The prediction of the course of minor psychiatric disorders. *Br. J. Psychiat.*, 135, 535–543

Keehn, R.J., Goldberg, I.D. and Beebe, G.W. (1974). Twenty-four year mortality follow-up of army veterans with disability separations for psychoneurosis in 1944. *Psychosom. Med.*, 36, 27–46

Malan, D. (1976). *The Frontier of Brief Psychotherapy. An Example of the Convergence of Research and Clinical Practice*, Plenum Publishing Corporation, New York

Malan, D.H., Heath, E.S., Bacal, H.A. and Balfour, F.H.G. (1975). Psychodynamic changes in untreated neurotic patients: 11 apparently genuine improvements. *Arch. gen. Psychiat.*, 32, 110–126

Mann, A.H., Jenkins, R. and Belsey, E. (1981). The twelve month outcome of patients with neurotic illness in general practice. Psychol. *Med.*, 11, 353–550

Moser, C.A. and Kalton, G. (1971). *Survey Methods in Social Investigation*, 2nd edn, Heinemann, London

Niskanen, P., Achte, K., Jaaskelainen, J., Karha, E. and Schroderus, M. (1974). *Psychiatric Fennica*, 339

Office of Population Censuses and Surveys (1980). *Mortality Statistics*, 1979, H.M.S.O., London

Oppenheim, A.M. (1966). *Questionnaire Design and Attitude Measurement*, Basic, London

Parloff, M.G., Waskow, I.E. and Wolfe, B.E. (1978). Research on therapist variables in relation to process and outcome. In: *Handbook of Psychotherapy and Behaviour Change: An Empirical Analysis* (Ed. Garfield, S.L. and Bergin, A.E.), 2nd edn, John Wiley, New York

Paykel, E.S., Prusoff, B.A. and Uhlenhuth, E.H. (1971). Scaling of life events. *Arch. gen. Psychiat.*, 25, 340–347

Ryle, A. (1975). *Frames and Cages*, Sussex University Press, London

Salmons, P.H. and Sims, A.C.P. (1981). Smoking profiles of patients admitted for neurosis. *Br. J. Psychiat.*, 139, 43–46

Scott, P.D. quoted in Goodwin, D.W., Guze, S.B. and Robins, E. (1969). Follow-up studies in obsessional neurosis. *Arch. gen. Psychiat.*, 20/2, 182–187

Sifneos, P.E. (1979). *Short Term Dynamic Psychotherapy: Evaluation and Technique*, Plenum Medical Book Company, London

Sims, A.C.P. (1973). The importance of a high tracing rate. *Lancet*, II, 433–435

Sims, A.C.P. (1974). An Investigation into Factors Predictive of the Prognosis in Neurosis: A Follow-up Study of Hospital Patients, Unpublished MD, University of Cambridge

Sims, A.C.P. and Gooding, K. (1975). The psychiatric outcome of 'normal' neurosis. *Br. J. Addict.*, 70, 33–40

Sims, A.C.P. (1975b). Factors predictive of outcome in neurosis. *Br. J. Psychiat.*, 127, 54-62

Sims, A.C.P. (1976). The consequences of severe neurosis. *Practitioner*, 216, 321-329

Sims, A.C.P. (1982). Towards the evaluation of treatment in neurosis. *J. psychiat. Treat. Eval.*; awaiting publication

Sims, A.C.P. and Gooding, K. (1975). The psychiatric outcome of 'normal' people at follow-up. *Psychiat. Res.*, 12, 167-175

Sims, A.C.P. and Prior, M.P. (1978). The pattern of mortality in severe neuroses. *Br. J. Psychiat.*, 133, 299-305

Sims, A.C.P. and Prior, M.P. (1982). Arteriosclerosis-related death in severe neurosis. *Comprehensive Psychiatry;* awaiting publication

Sims, A.C.P. and Rudge, B. (1979). Discriminators between neurotics who die and neurotics who live. *Acta Psychiat. Scand.*, 59, 317-325

Sloane, R.B., Staples, F.R., Cristol, A.H., Yorkston, N.J. and Whittal, K. (1975). *Psychotherapy Versus Behaviour Therapy*, Harvard University Press

Snaith, R.P., Bridges, G.W.K. and Hamilton, M. (1976). The Leeds Scales for the Self-Assessment of Anxiety and Depression. *Br. J. Psychiat.*, 128, 156-65

Strupp, H.H., Hadley, S.W. and Gomes-Schwartz, N. (1978). *Psychotherapy for Better or Worse; The Problem of Negative Effects*, Jason Aronson, New York

Strupp, H.H. and Hadley, S.W. (1979). Specific versus non-specific practices in psychotherapy. *Arch. gen. Psychiat.*, 36, 1125-36

Taylor, S.J.L.T. and Chave, S. (1964). *Mental Health and Environment*, Longmans, Green, London

Truax, C.B. and Carkhuff, R.R. (1967). *Toward Effective Counselling and Psychotherapy: Training & Practice*, Aldine, Chicago

Vázquez Barquero, J.L., Muñoz, P.E. and Madox Jaúregui, V. (1981). The interaction between physical illness and neurotic morbidity in the community. *Br. J. Psychiat.*, 139, 328-335

Wing, J.K., Cooper, J.E. and Sartorius, N. (1974). *The Measurement and Classification of Psychiatric Symptoms*, Cambridge University Press

Yalom, I.D. and Lieberman, M.A. (1971). A study of encounter group casualties. *Arch. gen. Psychiat.*, 25, 16-30

6 The Phenomena of Neurotic Illness

'In free air captive, in full day benighted,
I am as one for ever out of his element
Transparently enwombed, who from a bathysphere
Observes, wistful, amazed, but more affrighted,
Gay fluent forms of life weaving around
And dares not break the bubble and be drowned.'

C. Day Lewis, *The Neurotic*, 1948

In this chapter, I am embarking upon an impossible task. If all the novels and all the autobiographies that were ever written were combed for descriptions of neurotic pathology, there would still be much omitted. Many neurotics looking in these pages to see a picture of themselves will be disappointed. All I have been able to do is describe some of the commoner presentations.

Case Report

Mrs Theresa Kelly, aged 31, was referred to the hospital complaining of feeling acutely anxious, which prevented her going into crowds. She says she cannot relax on any occasion and cannot go shopping. Symptoms include difficulty in getting off to sleep, palpitations, sweating, overbreathing, and pins and needles of her arms and legs. She describes this, 'I feel as though I'm going to fall over; my head goes all funny'. She feels dizzy and unreal in some way. When these attacks occur she rushes out of her home into the garden. She is helped by talking to somebody. She is terrified that she will faint and be left lying in the street with nobody to look after her.

Theresa was born in Ireland. Foster parents, who had a son 10 years older than she, gave her a happy childhood but she felt she lacked normal parental love. At the age of 18 she started work as a nurse in Liverpool. On a visit home, she became pregnant by her long-term boyfriend; their baby was adopted. Two years later she married the father of her child and they had a further daughter a year later. She says that her husband was good and helpful, but she was irritable towards him, and they eventually separated. She now lives with her 5 year old daughter and does some part-time work.

In the past she has had surgery for a duodenal ulcer. Her first psychiatric treatment was with electro-convulsive therapy for 'depression' 7 years ago, and again 3 years later. She had had numerous physical symptoms in many different systems for the last 6 or 7 years.

Following her admission, when her husband came to visit her, she wrapped herself in a blanket and sat silently in the foetal position looking dejected. She became very agitated when she heard other patients claim that she was having a homosexual relationship on the ward. She complained of anaesthesia of parts of her face. Her hyperventilation attacks increased and she described seeing animals, for example, white mice running across the floor; she made a bed for the mice with her scarf. She answered nonsensically when asked questions and showed no concern about her illness. During a ward group she pointed out a rabbit jumping across the floor and giggled fatuously. Remembering this experience later she said that it was visible but she realised that it could not have happened.

What symptoms of neurosis did this patient show? There appears to have been sensory, motor and psychological symptoms of *hysteria;* the latter being of hysterical pseudo-dementia type with loss of memory for the period when they were experienced, visual hallucinations, mimicked buffoonery, disturbed behaviour; the whole episode provoked by a discreditable experience. At different times in the course of her illness, she had shown *phobic* symptoms, pathological *anxiety, hypochondriacal* ideas, *depersonalisation* and *neurotic depressive* symptoms. Depression was precipitated by the difficulties in looking after her child and the breakdown of the relationships with her husband. In fact, during the few weeks of her admission, she manifestated almost all the different types of neurotic reaction described later (table 1.3); she shows well the fluctuating nature of neurotic symptomatology. She had extreme difficulty in making relationships with members of staff and with other patients. As well as neurotic symptoms she had marked personality disorder. She was able to talk quite freely in large groups, but when it came to more intimate discussion with one other person, she would retreat into giggly bashfulness or morose depression, or alternatively produce more dramatic symptoms to prevent conversation. By the time of her discharge her symptoms had cleared, but problems in bringing up her child and in doing her work continued.

The Clinical Assessment of Neurotic Symptoms

We have gone to some length to show that what neurotic patients have in common is more important than the differences between them. Neurotic patients are different from other psychiatric patients, and also from people who are physically ill. In this chapter the emphasis is on the diversity of symptoms within neurosis. Before this, we will discuss how the doctor or therapist finds out how the patient feels using the method of empathy. The patient describes how he feels inside himself, and we understand this because we have had similar experiences in the past ('feeling dreadfully embarrassed, because people are looking at me'). Using our ability to put ourselves into the patient's situation, we question him to build up a picture of what it is like to be himself. Our aim in this is to understand his internal state well enough to be able to describe it to him and for him to recognise it as his own. This depends upon our ability to empathise and also upon our knowledge of the range of symptoms that occur.

We are concerned with his feelings and the way he sees his world, descriptively rather than analytically. That is, we are trying to obtain a detailed and insightful description of the patient's state rather than explaining what caused it to happen. This is the only rational starting place for trying to understand neurotic symptoms.

This empathic understanding of symptomatology must precede any type of psychotherapy. It is also an essential stage in valid psychiatric research, as it is the significance of events to the patient himself which is important. Jaspers (1962) has made the important distinction between thought and behaviour that is understandable to an outside observer, and what is ultimately understandable. Psychotic thinking is, in these terms, ultimately not understandable. Neurotic thinking and behaviour, however inappropriate and socially unacceptable, is in fact ultimately understandable. That is, when the doctor talks with his patient in detail and understands the background which has led up to this particular behaviour, he is able to say, 'If I had been in those circumstances, with that past experience and this particular way of looking at life, I can understand how I could have carried out this particular action'.

Self-experience in Neurosis

Neurotic conflicts about self may be revealed in chronic low self-esteem, or anxious over-involvement with self. The person may devalue himself, assuming that he will be unable to cope with the demands made upon him, or he may crave attention and appreciation. The very emphasis he puts upon his own self-interest precludes the possibility of a mutually rewarding relationship with others. This anxious or deprecating awareness of self may include disordered ideas about his body; dislike and contempt for his own body, distortion of the way he sees it, or excessive concern about appearance or health (figure 6.1). It may be generalised, affecting the whole of the way he sees himself and his body or it may be localised, affecting individual organs or parts of the body; for example, the woman who feels that she has an atrociously ugly nose.

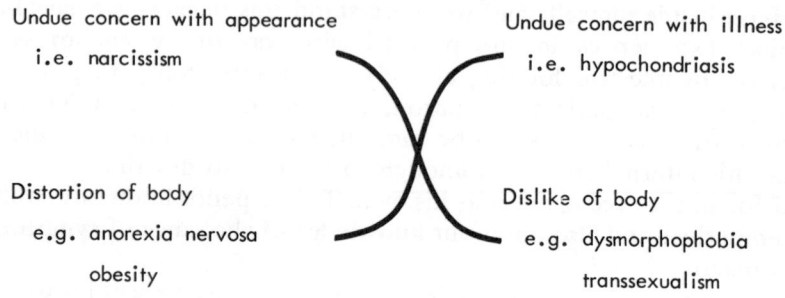

Undue concern with appearance
i.e. narcissism

Undue concern with illness
i.e. hypochondriasis

Distortion of body
e.g. anorexia nervosa
obesity

Dislike of body
e.g. dysmorphophobia
transsexualism

Figure 6.1   Body image disorders

Fundamental to the experience of self is the distinction between what is self and what is not self. A healthy person makes assumptions about himself, so that he can function efficiently without needing to introspect. These assumptions are; a capacity for activity, awareness of unity, a sense of identity and a knowledge of the definition of self.

Activity of self implies that I do something and know that I am doing it deliberately. The neurotic may feel himself to be incapable of effective action, and feel that what actions he does undertake, although carried out by himself, are imposed upon him by pressure from outside circumstances. This is quite different from the belief in outside control, 'passivity', of the schizophrenic. The neurotic may believe that his own behaviour is inevitable; the schizophrenic that it is not his own behaviour at all.

The second quality is *unity;* that is, 'I am aware that I am one person'. This does not imply that a normal person can never be inconsistent, is always predictable, rational or predetermined. The personality has many manifestations which can express itself in a variety of ways according to circumstances. So a normal person will have masculine and feminine aspects, can be passive or aggressive, rationalistic or aesthetic, and so on. Despite this range of possible manifestations, the person knows himself to be a single whole and the different parts of himself are components and not separate entities. Neurotic conflict can be such a divisive force that this integrity of the self may be in doubt to the patient himself. The neurotic experience of 'the double phenomenon' will be described in more detail later in the chapter; not infrequently the neurotic feels different parts of himself in conflict with each other to such an extent *as if* he were more than one person.

Identity is the quality of continuity; that is what I was in the past I still am. The neurotic may feel that at some particular time in the past he radically changed for the worse due to circumstances outside his control, that his capacity for coping was altered by this experience, and that he is not, and now never will be, as competent as he used to be. To the ouside observer this response may seem out of proportion. Again, the neurotic's experience of lack of continuity is quite different from psychotic experience. The psychotic may believe himself to be a different person, whereas the neurotic believes himself to be irretrievably deteriorated but still the same person. Often neurotics are concerned about their identity in the sense that they do not know where they belong in relation to other people.

The final quality is *definition;* that is I know where I end and the outside world begins. A schizophrenic patient may have a blurring of the margins of self, believing that his thoughts can influence someone miles away or that harmful rays are eating his body, but the neurotic experience of lack of definition is different from this. In neurosis, it is not that he mistakes the boundaries of self and ascribes to the outside world in a delusional sense what is going on inside himself; it is more a loss of the feeling of capacity for self to influence the outside world.

What then is neurotic experience of self? The neurotic does not have the capacity to accept himself and feel reasonably comfortable, neither does he feel confident in judging his own capabilities. Knowing quite precisely what a person can expect of himself is important for success in any human endeavour. This, associated with appropriate self-esteem and maintaining consistent goals to be achieved, often is lacking in the neurotic. He does not know what he can hope to achieve and therefore attempts either nothing or the unattainable.

A girl, aged 22, had been treated in a day hospital for most of the last 4 years. She had reasonable 'A' level passes from school but no further educational attainments. She applied to several colleges to train as a social worker, and when rejected she became very upset refusing to consider any other work less demanding of a good health record.

There is always a discrepancy between the way a person sees himself, how others see him and what he is actually like; the neurotic cannot tolerate this disparity. His goals are fluctuating and inconsistent, not maintained over time, and sometimes unattainable. He finds himself uncomfortable to live with. He describes either an inability to cope, or coping but with extreme difficulty. He comes to regard himself as a non-coper and this produces feelings of self-disgust. He may describe this in terms of hating himself, and he may show a variety of symptoms, both psychological and physical, which demonstrates his feelings of low self-esteem. At the same time, this concern about himself, whether others value him, and his anxiety over his capacity to cope makes the neurotic a self-centred person.

The *affect of helplessness* has been described in chapter 4 as occurring in life-settings in which illness develops; a situation which has been called the giving-up given-up complex. Where the patient is threatened with loss or separation and is experiencing great difficulty with coping, discouragement, despair, giving up or depression may be described. The characteristics were listed by Engel (1968) as follows:

(1)   The affect of helplessness and hopelessness; the patient describes himself as being at the end of his tether, unable to cope and not knowing which way to turn. He talks about giving up and being incapable of any action to resolve his dilemma.
(2)   There is a loss of self-esteem; he feels himself no longer to be competent or in control, he may feel himself to be damaged, maimed or mutilated.
(3)   There is a loss of gratification in his relationships and roles in life. He may express dissatisfaction with his marriage, his job and he feels a failure to achieve his ambitions.
(4)   There is a disruption of the normal sense of continuity between the past, present and future. The future seems bleak and hopeless.
(5)   There is a painful remembering of times when his self-esteem and sense of well-being was lowered; this reactivation of memory especially concerns past failures and embarrassments, and also griefs and loss.

Prominent in how the neurotic feels about himself is disordered mood. Depression is associated with feelings of low self-esteem, helplessness and hopelessness. Anxiety is also commonly experienced and relates to feelings and fears of loss of self and loss of status. The neurotic's anxious need for appreciation arises from the fear which is near the surface, that his status and even his existence is threatened, and that unless he asserts himself he will lose what little he has left. The neurotic shows his low self-esteem in anger directed at himself; he is frustrated at himself for this failure to cope and hates himself. There is often a mood of self-reference. He feels an object of adverse attention, that he sticks out like a sore thumb, and he feels embarrassed and sensitive.

Irritability is such a common feature of neuroses that Snaith (1981) has asked why there is no category in the International Classification of 'irritability neurosis'. This emotion may be shown in verbal or physical acts of aggression; the patient, more often female, shouts or criticises, throws cups or other handy domestic objects, slams doors and is generally unable to control an intense feeling of internal tension. The mood is usually associated with misery and low self-esteem, and often followed by remorse. Those closest to the patient, especially husband and children, are especially likely to be the target of her impulsiveness. It may be cyclical, associated with premenstrual tension (Tonks, 1975). Irritability may, paradoxically, be increased by anxiolytic drugs such as the benzodiazepines rather than reduced. Psychiatrists make a clear distinction between the symptoms described to them of anxiety, depression and irritability. However, these symptoms are much less clearly differentiated according to patients who do not usually distinguish depression from anxiety (Leff, 1978).

Feeling himself to be two (or more) quite different personalities has been described in neurosis. On close enquiry this does not have the elements of a psychotic disturbance. There are no delusions nor hallucinations, and the neurotic is attempting to describe the conflicts inside himself. This neurotic phenomenon of the 'double' bears a close relationship to the north European myth of the 'wraith' (or doppelganger); that is, the situation in which the person, just before he dies, sees himself carrying out all the most reprehensible acts of his life. It is this neurotic conflict which is depicted in *The Double* by Dostoievski, or *Dr. Jekyll and Mr. Hyde* by R.L. Stevenson.

Some patients find that they can only explain the extreme inconsistency between their behaviour and their aspirations by considering themselves to be two entirely different people. According to Morton Prince (1905), 'Nearly all writers of fiction and even biographers have failed to recognise — what in these modern days the most advanced criminologists and penologists have recognised — that man is a many sided creature and woman, if I may venture to say it, particularly so. No one is wholly good or wholly bad; or wholly hard or wholly sentimental . . . according as which side is uppermost will a person appear to his neighbours and to the world as a person of this kind of character or that kind'. This divergence of the 'many sides' may in extreme form result in multiple personality where different personalities, sometimes oblivious of each other, lead independent lives in the same individual.

Depersonalisation is very commonly experienced by neurotic patients; they have great difficulty in describing the symptom. In depersonalisation the ordinary feelings of familiarity concerning oneself are lost or altered, whereas in derealisation the feelings of familiarity for what is outside self are altered. These symptoms commonly occur together. Although the patient may describe the symptom in perceptual terms, 'everything looks a long way away', it is not a true disturbance of perception but of mood. The patient is aware that the change he experiences is subjective. He may feel himself, or parts of himself to be unreal, remote, flat, lifeless, automatic, changed qualitatively in such a way as to lose part of its essence. Depersonalisation is intimately associated with the way the neurotic sees himself. It is a feeling of loss of self, always associated with unpleasant emotion.

A divorced woman, aged 30, was seen in a medical ward following overdosage. She describe the emotional component of her loneliness and depersonalisation: 'I felt as if I didn't fit into the world . . . When I saw the snow, I felt I couldn't cope. One day it wasn't there and the next it was. I saw it and it upset me and I went to pieces . . . I felt I did not want to be alive because I was not related to anything. I just seemed totally out of everything and I started to cry. I couldn't cope with the hurt and the pain. I felt I never would feel part of anything'.

Bodily Symptoms

Physical complaints are a prominent part of many neurotic syndromes. Dissatisfaction with bodily shape or appearance (dysmorphophobia) has been described earlier in this chapter. This usually takes the form of an overvalued idea, in which a part of the body (nose, breasts, etc.) is disliked; the sufferer feels that other people are noticing it, and commenting adversely upon it; it may come to be the dominating thought in the person's life to the exclusion of all enjoyment, and all practical and useful pursuits. Hay (1970) studied 45 people who were assessed before cosmetic surgery for the nose. He found that 26 of these were basically normal people with a neurotic reaction; nine showed evidence of personality disorder of moderate degree; another nine suffered from severe personality disorder, and one patient was psychotic.

The physical symptoms of hypochondriasis, hysteria and deliberate disability are shown to be linked in figure 6.2 (p.122) as different instances of 'illness behaviour'; that is, the behaviour appropriate to physical illness without such organic disorder being present. Conversion symptoms of hysteria may involve almost any organ, and would appear to be associated with the positive gains in the patient's life situation that result from his being ill, and regarded as so by other people. Hypochondriacal symptoms result from fear of illness, or misinterpretation of the normal sensorium, or minor symptoms as being evidence of serious, and perhaps lethal, illness. In both hysteria and hypochondriasis the patient's interest and concern is concentrated upon the physical symptoms, and not upon the supposed psychological causes.

Anxiety has two components — psychological experience and

physical symptoms. The somatic symptoms are autonomic in nature. The psychological response of arousal with anxiety results in these physical manifestations, which are experienced as frightening in themselves, thus increasing the arousal and anxiety; the interplay of physical and psychological symptoms tends towards exacerbation.

Sleep disorder is prominent in neuroses. Typically this is an exaggeration of the response a normal person has to the stress and conflict of a difficult day. Rehearsing the problems and frustrations of the day and dwelling on its insults and injuries produces such a state of arousal that sleep becomes impossible. Typically the neurotic patient has difficulty in getting off to sleep; he wakes at times during the night, and is less satisfied with the quality of his sleep than the healthy person. In an electroencephalographic comparison of the sleep of neurotic patients with normal subjects, Jovanovic (1978) found that the neurotic patients had more wakefulness in the first third of the night. Although the two groups were asleep for the same mean length of time, the neurotics spent more time lying awake in bed, and awoke during the night more frequently. The neurotic patients spent a shorter time in deep sleep and there was a longer period of time before their first episode of REM (rapid eye movement) sleep. The sleep of neurotic subjects was impaired by unfamiliar surroundings to a greater extent than normal subjects.

Experience of Relationships

Neuroticism catalyses all that is disruptive in human relationships. Attitudes and ways of seeing oneself vitally affect relating to others. The way he thinks about his past relationships with people, the way they treat him, and what he felt able to communicate to them are affected by neurotic attitudes. Present relationships and also making plans for relationships in the future are affected. All areas of social life are dominated by neurotic thinking: work, marriage, home and family relationships, and external affairs including public position, economic matters and relationships with the law.

Self is always viewed in relation to others; how one sees oneself is not dependent so much upon other people's opinion but upon what one believes other people's opinion to be. It is in this sense that the word *sensitive* is used in psychiatry. A young woman with Crohn's disease had lost a lot of weight and had a very poor appetite. She hated herself so thin, felt she could not buy any new clothes and did not like to go out in the streets because she did not want people to see her so ugly; she was sensitive. The capacity to develop social relationships occurs through various stages from childhood to adult life, and at each stage it is related to the way the person views himself. The ability to relate is vitally connected therefore with feelings of self-esteem.

Manipulativeness is not confined to neurosis; in one sense all human relationships are manipulative. However, in successful relationship, this is rewarding both to the manipulator and to the recipient, and is not intrinsically sinister. The chief characteristic of neurotic manipulation is that it is unsuccessful for subject and object alike. The neurotic fails to achieve his goals because they are unrealistic, and the means he uses are destructive. A special case is, of course, when two people relate both of them using neurotic mechanisms. Sometimes their very neuroticism and shared need for dependence may be a factor in sustaining the relationship.

The neurotic characteristic of difficulty with coping manifests itself also in relationships. The neurotic shows no confidence in his ability to manage relationships and is socially inept. This may be a general characteristic, or only revealed in certain circumstances, for example, the person who fails to get on with a succession of employers. The difficulty he has in sustaining realistic goals impairs relationships. He makes unreasonable and excessive demands of the other person so they feel him either to be importunate like a child, or smothering like an over-protective parent. He also has difficulty in conveying what his expectations of the relationship are to the other person.

Neurotic decision-making also affects relationships. Because of his previous experience based on his previous neurotic behaviour, and because of his current neurotic attitudes, his ability to make successful choices is seriously impaired; these unsatisfactory choices will lead to further difficulties in the future. His indecisiveness and lack of confidence in his ability to choose is understandably based upon his lack of success in making satisfactory decisions in the past. This is related to 'the neurotic paradigm' described in chapter 5. It is also related to the model of neurosis described as *learned help-lessness*. The neurotic has learned a method of coping which is unsatisfactory and leads to further problems, he feels that it is inevitable that he will carry out further behaviour, make further choices that will inevitably lead to further difficulties in relationships. The neurotic will also have difficulties in relationships because of his inability to control and use his feelings of aggression appropriately. This is a quite frequent explanation for the neurotic mother's impulsive abuse of her child following other frustrations in her life.

The Neurotic Syndromes

Anxiety States

It would be maladaptive not to experience anxiety under some circumstances; it is a necessary part of the response of the organism to external stress. Anxiety can be assessed in terms of whether the emotion is appropriate, or pathological in its origin, intensity and duration. When it is not attributable to real threat, or persists after the danger has been removed, it has become pathological. Psychiatrists make a clear distinction between the subjective experiences of depression and anxiety. However, neurotic patients suffering these emotions are not nearly so sure that they can distinguish between them. They do, however, make a clear distinction between anxiety and irritability. An anxiety state may occur at any age; it is commoner in females than males. The two major types of provocation for anxiety are fear of separation and fear of the unknown or danger.

The experience of anxiety as an unpleasant, subjective emotion can be contrasted with its objective, somatic manifestations. Frequently psychological and somatic anxiety occur synchronously, but this may not necessarily be the case. A person may feel anxious and yet have few somatic indications, and vice versa. A third component is the behavioural; carrying out behaviour associated with anxiety, for example, running away. Various words are used to describe the feelings of anxiety — tension, worry, apprehensiveness, nervousness, fretting, uneasiness, concern, and expressions such as 'needle' and 'butterflies in the stomach' are used to describe anxiety in specific situations. The somatic symptoms of anxiety are associated with arousal of the sympathetic, autonomic nervous system. The subject experiences palpitations, dry mouth, dilatation of the pupils, panting, shortness of breath, sweating with pallor of skin (a cold sweat), anorexia and gastro-intestinal discomfort, abdominal churning, choking or feeling tight in the throat, trembling and dizziness.

Anxiety may be persistent or occur in panic attacks. These latter are discrete episodes of extreme somatic anxiety, whilst in between attacks the person may feel mildly anxious or quite normal. In a panic attack there are often clear precipitating circumstances which produce initial intense feelings of anxiety in the patient. Overbreathing is often prominent, and by reducing the partial pressure of carbon dioxide in the blood, secondary symptoms of paraesthesiae (pins and needles) in the limbs, dizziness, faintness, and eventually tetany, occur. These frightening symptoms increase the anxiety, and so the momentum of attack increases. It usually ends with the patient lying down, or alternatively, rushing into fresh air, gasping; conscious, but often with a depersonalisation experience. The attack may last for less than a minute or up to a few hours, but usually for about a quarter of an hour. It may occur infrequently or several times a day.

Unlike phobic states in which anxiety is situational, free-floating anxiety occurs in anxiety neurosis without specific precipitants. It is not always easy to make the distinction between anxiety state, and the trait of anxiety as a feature of the 'affective personality disorder'. The latter is characteristic of 'chronic worriers' who show this as a permanent feature of their personality.

Anxiety often accompanies hysteria, depressive neurosis, obsessive-compulsive neurosis, phobic states, or depersonalisation. When anxiety is experienced with one of these other neurotic illnesses, diagnosis is usually assigned to the other condition. Tension, agitation, frustration and irritability are frequent psychological concomitants with the symptom of anxiety. Anxiety state is not a unitary diagnosis but describes many different presentations of symptoms of different types.

Anxiety neurosis may begin at any age but first attacks are commonest in young adults, especially those predisposed with anxious or 'anankastic personality'. The attack often occurs with stress factors, for example, following real or perceived danger, or more commonly, conflict situations especially where the patient finds himself in an ambiguous situation, frustrated from any effective action, and is exposed to public scrutiny and disapproval. Anxiety neurosis may start with frequent panic attacks or generalised free-floating anxiety. Anxiety may be experienced only in social situations, especially when the person feels himself criticised. It is not uncommon for the source of anxiety to be displaced, as in the case of a girl who had a quite unjustified fear that she had developed venereal disease and was acutely anxious, but had in fact two years previously been treated for Hodgkins disease about which she claimed to be unconcerned.

Anxiety states may be of acute onset and limited duration, or they may continue with varying severity for many years. Patients often describe anxiety and depression together. Anxiety may occur prodromally in a depressive illness, schizophrenia or organic conditions such as senile dementia. Anxiety symptoms often occur with physical illness, either as a symptom of the illness, or as part of the emotional reaction to it. For example, hyperthyroidism is frequently difficult to distinguish from anxiety state.

Hysteria

Hysteria is defined in the 9th Revision of the International Classification of Diseases as follows: 'Mental disorders in which motives, of which the patient seems unaware, produce either a restriction of the field of consciousness or disturbances of motor or sensory function which may seem to have psychological advantage or symbolic value. It may be characterised by conversion phenomena or dissociative phenomena. In the conversion form the chief or only symptoms consists of psychogenic disturbance of function in some part of the body, e.g. paralysis, tremor, blindness, deafness, seizures. In the dissociative variety, the most prominent feature is a narrowing of the field of consciousness which seems to serve an unconscious purpose and is commonly accompanied or followed by a selective amnesia. There may be dramatic but essentially superficial changes of personality sometimes taking the form of a fugue (wandering state). Behaviour may mimic psychosis or rather the patient's idea of psychosis'.

A student nurse, aged 19, was planning to go on holiday with some friends to Israel. She came from a small market town, had never been abroad before and had never flown in an aeroplane. About a week before the flight she developed paralysis of her left arm; there was 'glove' anaesthesia, reflexes were preserved, tone was flaccid; there was no muscle wasting or fasciculation and no other neurological signs. The general practitioner who looked after nursing staff referred her to a neurologist who admitted her for investigation. He felt the risk of letting her go on holiday was too great, and advised her to cancel her flight. Her symptoms cleared up completely within a fortnight. No other provoking stress was found. At 18 months follow-up she remained symptom free.

There are few diagnostic categories in psychiatry where there is more disagreement than over hysteria (Lewis, 1975). Different authors have included quite different groups of symptoms, and yet the category is still useful. Chodoff and Lyons (1958) have listed five senses in which hysteria is commonly used: (1) a behavioural pattern habitually exhibited by individuals with hysterical personalities; (2) conversion reactions and dissociative states; (3) a psychosomatic disorder complicating abnormal personalities, resulting in anxieties and phobias; (4) particular psychopathological content operating at an unconscious level; and (5) a term of opprobrium. Slater (1965) carried out a follow-up study of patients' diagnosed hysteria in a neurological hospital and found a very large number had been rediagnosed as having serious physical or psychiatric illness at follow-up. He recommended abandoning the term. Perley and Guze (1962) have described a poly-symptomatic condition which really bears very little relation to the definition of hysteria above. This, Briquet's syndrome, has been used as a synonym for hysteria but is actually a description of severe chronic neurosis of mixed type with an emphasis upon hypochondriasis. Hysteria and hypo-chondriacal neurosis are probably best considered as different forms of 'illness behaviour' (Mechanic, 1966); that is, the symptoms or behaviour of organic illness occur without physical disease being present. This is represented in figure 6.2.

An hysterical reaction may be found secondary to other physical or psychiatric illness; that is an inappropriate, unsuccessful way of coping with conflict, the cause of which, in this case, is the other illness. From the diagnostic point of view, it is very important to identify the underlying illness, rather than being satisfied only with the identification of secondary hysteria. For example, hysterical symptoms presenting in a patient over the age of 40 for the first time should not be accepted at face value. An underlying cause in terms of another illness should be expected. Hysterical symptoms may be manifested as a secondary reaction to a depressive illness, to organic states, for example, following head injury or in the early stages of dementia, with epilepsy, and not infrequently, mental handicap. Hysterical symptoms in these conditions are similar to those in primary hysteria but it is, of course, very important to diagnose the underlying condition.

Hysterical symptoms may occur at any age, in childhood as well as in adult life (Merskey, 1979). However they are much more common in females than males; it used to be thought they did not occur in males. They occur most frequently round about the time of puberty, and first occurrence becomes less frequent after that age.

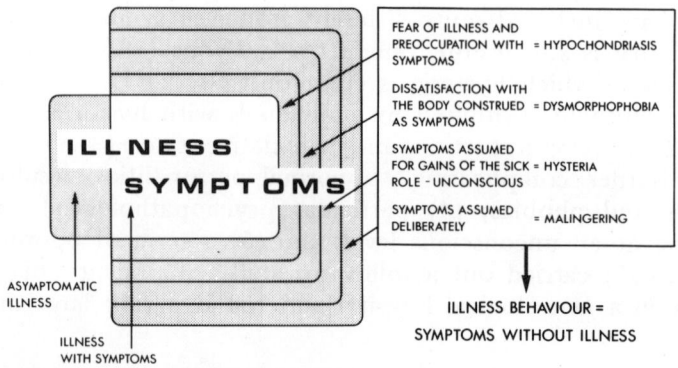

Figure 6.2   Illness and illness behaviour

Hysterical symptoms in a young girl have a benign prognosis. However, the older the age of the patient, and the longer the course of illness, the less satisfactory is the outcome. Most commonly there is a major psychological conflict present at the onset of symptoms. This may be concerned with the thought of physical or psychological illness in the patient, but more often is associated with emotional conflict or an acute problem with relationships. Characteristic of such precipitating factors was the girl aged 18, who developed hysterical disturbance of gait when she fell in love with a boy to whom her family objected.

Conversion symptoms are those where there is a psychogenic disturbance of function in some part of the body, for example, there may be paralysis, tremor, blindness, deafness or seizure. *Dissociative* symptoms demonstrate a narrowing of the field of consciousness, and this is usually associated with amnesia. It is quite common for the paralysis to be partial in nature: a patient was hampered from walking quickly for any distance by an inability to move her foot at the ankle joint. It is a usual finding with hysterical symptoms that they have a marked effect upon social relationships with significant people; they have psychological advantage or symbolic value, for example, relieving her of obligations. They allow her to retire from competitive situations in life, but she may lead an active life 'bravely coping with her difficulties'.

The overlap between hysterical symptoms and anxiety is important. Often the patient denies feeling anxious but on physiological assessment, measures of somatic anxiety may be increased beyond that found in anxiety states. Occasionally the onset of hysterical symptoms occurs during acute panic, especially a dissociative fugue state. A schoolteacher found himself in a city in which the signs in the shops were in French. He did not know where he was and could not remember how he got there. In fact he had received a criminal charge at his home in Birmingham, U.K. and had flown to Montreal, for both of which he claimed complete amnesia.

There may be overlap between hysterical and depressive or obsessional neurosis; the latter is particularly difficult to treat, 'La belle indifference' is a frequent mood of hysteria, in which the patient shows a lack of concern with her symptoms or accepts them with surprising placidity in view of such severe disability in a young person. It is, however, not a consistent finding in hysteria, and is difficult to evaluate, but occasionally it is very obvious, and lends support to the idea of 'secondary gain'; that is, there are unconscious but real advantages accruing from the symptoms. There may, on the contrary, be quite a marked degree of depression in association with the hysterical symptoms and this, of course, makes the diagnosis more difficult. On other occasions there appears to be considerable anger which the patient may find difficult to express, but which may take the form of concealed animosity towards relations or staff of the hospital.

The course of the condition may be continuous or episodic. Subsequent episodes may involve the same part of the body, but quite frequently elsewhere. A patient had hysterical loss of use of an arm at the age of 15 and then hysterical dissociation showing altered consciousness, *approximate answers* with amnesia at the age of 20, having been completely free of symptoms in between. By *approximate answers* is meant the situation in which the respondent just fails to get the answers to questions correct—'How many legs has a cow?' 'Five'. Psychosis is rare following an hysterical illness; depression is more common. There is an increased suicide rate for female patients with hysteria, and there is also a marked increase of death from accidents. Most uncomplicated conversion symptoms carry a benign prognosis, especially when they occur once at an early age, associated with clear conflict and begin to respond to simple measures such as physiotherapy.

Hysteria needs to be distinguished from hysterical personality disorder. The two may coexist, but the majority of people who develop hysteria do not have hysterical premorbid personality. Hysterical symptoms may develop under stress, in people of such personality, but equally other neurotic symptoms, for example, depressive neurosis may occur in a person with hysterical personality.

Various tests can be used to distinguish hysteria from other conditions. These depend upon the nature of the conversion or dissociative symptom; for example, neurological examination or tests of vision or hearing may reveal the abnormality to be quite unphysiological. The characteristic 'corkscrew' visual field chart for hysterical restriction of vision is shown in figure 6.3. There is

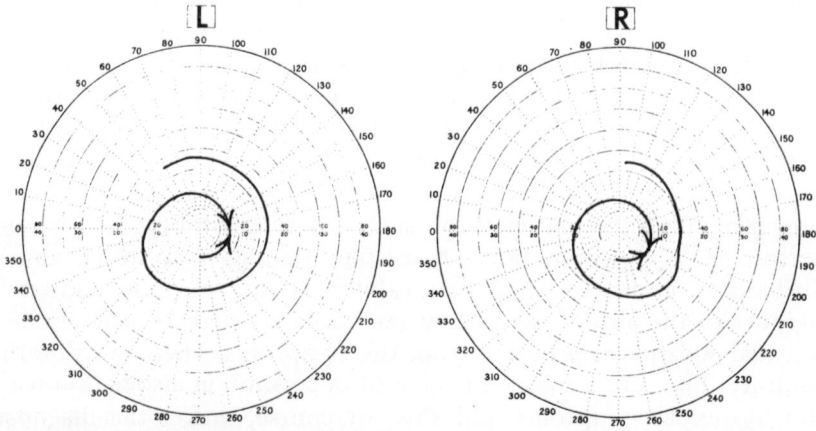

Figure 6.3   Visual field in hysteria

no way in which this spiral could occur with an organic disturbance of vision, as it implies the visual field changing over a few minutes. This patient, a young man, had been hit on the head with a sword which lacerated his left ear. Two weeks later he complained that he could not see properly. No other abnormality was found on careful examination.

'Hysteria' encompasses various other syndromes, unusual symptoms and manifestations of distress such as Munchausen Syndrome, Ganser Syndrome, compensation neurosis, multiple personality, and mass hysteria. In Munchausen or the 'Hospital Addiction' syndrome, serious illness is simulated by the patient who achieves repeated hospital admissions (124 in one of the series described by Barker, 1962) and multiple operations. They are usually isolated, dependent people who require emotional support but because of their incompetence in human relationships can only relate to institutions and not to individuals. Ganser's syndrome (1898) is a form of dissociation characterised by the giving of approximate answers, clouding of consciousness, recent history of physical or emotional stress and amnesia for the period during which the symptoms occurred. Compensation neurosis must be distinguished from traumatic neurosis where neurotic symptoms occur in reaction to the stress of the event (for example, anxiety following road accident), or malingering where symptoms are assumed deliberately and consciously (Trimble, 1981). Compensation neurosis occurs when symptoms are acquired or prolonged unconsciously in association with likely compensation. Epidemic hysteria is described in chapter 8.

Multiple personality is a condition that has been of special interest to psychiatrists in the past. Morton Prince (1905) described in detail the case of Miss Beecham, and reported twenty such cases. He clearly recognised the hysterical origins of the different personalities; however, it is now clear that the intense interest of doctors in such cases has often prompted patients to produce yet more exotic symptoms; that is, multiple personality is largely iatrogenic in origin (Slater and Roth, 1969). Miss Beecham showed four different personalities; most of these were not aware of the others existence, but one called Sally used to tease and persecute the other personalities and, in fact, try to harm them.

A relationship with those responsible for treatment that is friendly and accepting but not hostile or theatrical, is likely to carry a better prognosis. There is an increased risk of suicide and also of death from accidents, especially in female hysterics; there is also increased risk of dependence upon alcohol, upon psychotropic drugs and also upon institutions and other people. The long term prognosis is usually that the symptoms remit but there may be residual neurotic symptoms and further episodes of hysteria or other neurotic condition. Some few patients manifest hysterical symptoms over a long time and may develop permanent physical disability.

Phobic States

Phobias are unreasonable fears, or 'neurotic states with abnormally intense dread of certain objects or specific situations which would not normally have that affect' (WHO, 1977). There is considerable over-lap with anxiety, and when anxiety spreads from a specific provo-cation more generally it is considered to be an anxiety rather than a phobic state. Subjectively phobias take the form of situational anxiety; anxiety associated with specific circumstances or objects, as represented in table 6.1. Anxiety-prone traits, or consistent behavioural characteristics of the individual, are described in chapter 7 with personality disorders. Phobic states have been classified by Marks (1970) into animal phobias and agoraphobias, 'if ever we are tempted to think that all phobic states are unity which reflects the same disorder and aetiology, we can quickly dispel this illusion simply by looking at the startling contrast between animal phobias and agoraphobias. These two conditions differ radically in onset, course, symptomatology, response to treatment and psychophysiological measures'.

Agoraphobia, etymologically the fear of the market place, is the occurrence of recurrent anxiety on going into a busy public place. Sufferers feel that they will become conspicuous by collapsing in public, and other people will notice them. As they become increas-ingly concerned under these circumstances, the somatic symptoms

Table 6.1 *Anxiety and phobic conditions*

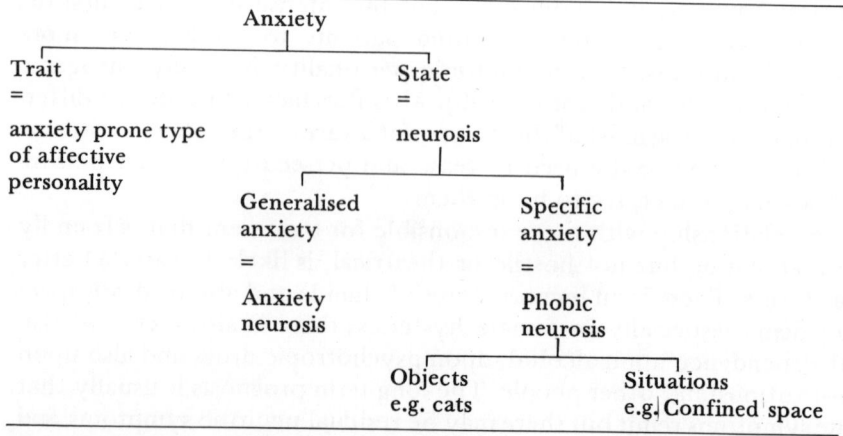

of anxiety occur. They become dizzy with hyperventilation, and feel that they might faint or fall over, which increases their panic. Eventually phobic symptoms prevent their sufferers entering certain situations altogether; such a person may stop going to an enclosed shopping arcade, or her fear of cats may prevent her visiting relations. This may generalise to such an extent that the individual is unable to go out of the house beyond the garden gate. She may feel able to travel with somebody else whom she knows well, or be at home if there is someone else there; this may result in a phobic housewife keeping her husband off work, or children off school. Fear of being with other people in a busy situation may result in difficulty in travelling on buses or trains. The patient is terrified that she may suddenly feel ill, and want to get off the bus but be unable to do so. Such a person may deliberately take a bus that makes frequent stops, rather than the express.

Recently, *space phobia* has been described (Marks, 1981), as a distinct entity from agoraphobia. In an account of 13 patients, with symptoms superficially similar to agoraphobia, he pointed out four distinctive features of space phobia: average age 55, whilst for agoraphobics it was 25; fears of falling in an open space rather than of the 'market' itself; less satisfactory response to behavioural treatment; frequently, evidence of organic disease of the brain or cardiovascular system. Whether or not this really is a distinct syndrome, it emphasises the importance of full physical examination and exclusion of organic conditions in patients who are thought to be neurotic.

Claustrophobia is fear of being in an enclosed space. In practice, it is not clearly distinct from agoraphobia, as the most common enclosed space of which people are afraid is the one where there are other people present, for example, a department store, church or concert hall. The sufferer often gains some reassurance from sitting near the back so that he can rush out. However, very often the fear will prevent him going into anxiety provoking situations.

The variety of situations from which people may become phobic is very large. However, fear of embarrassment is a frequent component. A 25-year-old married secretary had a great fear that she would suddenly need to pass urine at an inconvenient time. She would get this fear during a telephone call if it seemed that it was likely to last a long time. If she tried to go to a shop 100 yards from her office during the lunch break, she often had the urge to micturate on reaching the door of the shop. She would rush back to her office only to realise the urge had gone. Her journey from home to work in the morning took 40 minutes including a journey by train. She would make 10 visits to different public toilets during this time.

Phobias may occur for animals or parts of animals, for example, feathers. They may generalise from animals to all furry objects, or from a dislike of cats to all situations in which the person might see a cat. There is usually a reasonable basis for the object attracting some fear, or at least anxiety, but for the phobic patient this fear has got out of proportion and it limits his ability to lead a normal life. Such a common, and in some ways understandable fear, taken to grossly exaggerated lengths was described by a patient, aged 40, who had seen numerous plastic surgeons and psychiatrists because she had complained for the last 20 years of a furrowed forehead. She was terrified of looking like her mother whom she felt was prematurely aged. She spent 5-6 hours a day making herself up to obscure any wrinkles and she looked in the mirror about 40 times a day. She talked about her great fear of growing old.

Phobic conditions sometimes have their origins in childhood; an unpleasant happening occurring fortuitously at the same time as contact with the situation for which the person subsequently becomes phobic. Alternatively they may develop gradually, the person becoming anxious about going out, or going shopping, especially when her ability to go out is restricted, for example, by being at home looking after young children — the so-called housebound housewife. Phobic states are commoner in females than males but occur in both sexes. They commonly have their onset in the early twenties.

Obsessive-Compulsive Disorders

These are conditions in which the most prominent symptom is a repetitive feeling of subjective compulsion, which cannot be got rid of, to carry out some action, to dwell upon an idea, to recall an experience or to ruminate on an abstract topic. At the same time the patient feels that this obsession should be resisted. The unwanted thoughts which intrude, the insistency of words or ideas, ruminations or trains of thought, are perceived by the patient on reflection to be inappropriate or senseless. The obsessional idea is recognised both as alien to the person's nature, but also as coming from inside himself. The word *obsession* is often reserved for ideas, and *compulsion* for behaviour.

Common amongst obsessional ideas are repetitive checking or counting of numbers, or saying words or phrases in the head; 'the British Socialist Party', or 'I must remember what Father would have done'. Numerical obsessions may involve elaborate calculations which, if any errors occur, have to be started again from the beginning. Ruminations may take the form of repetitive worries or elaborate fantasies always following a similar pattern, sometimes of an antisocial, blasphemous or criminal nature; frequently also philosophical. The connection between thoughts and actions is often involved in obsessive-compulsive disorder; for example, the priest may be tortured by the obsessional idea that he will utter a blasphemy in church; the mother worries continually about sticking a pin in her baby; a patient washes her hands compulsively fifty times a day because of her fear of dirt. Sometimes ruminative fantasies can be quite obscure; a girl had a repetitive rumination in which she imagined herself to be an banana — she found this fantasy both frightening and irresistible.

It has often been considered that rituals are formed in order to relieve anxiety, for example, obsessive repeated washing of hands to try and cleanse from contamination, and this to assuage guilt, as Lady Macbeth. Resisting the obsessional ritual or attempting to prevent the obsessional thoughts would then lead to increased anxiety. However, Beech (1974) has commented that there are many obsessionals whose anxiety is not relieved by carrying out the compulsive act or thinking the obsessional thought, rather anxiety increases on these occasions and is diminished by successfully arresting the obsession. It is, therefore, difficult to see what function the obsession serves.

Like other neurotic reactions, obsessive-compulsive symptoms may manifest secondary to conflict, or to physical illness, or to another psychiatric condition. Obsessional symptoms may occur with anxiety state and other neurotic disorders; they are also quite frequent in the early stages of a depressive illness, in schizophrenia with the bizarre colouring characteristic of that disorder, and in organic states. It is sometimes difficult to distinguish the repetitive ritualistic behaviour that occurs in epilepsy and some other organic conditions from obsessional neurosis. However, an important quality of the latter is the patient's subjective feeling of a need to resist the symptoms.

Obsessional ideas and compulsive rituals are a prominent part of the games and learning experiences of young children, and certainly not pathological. Obsessional symptoms first occur commonly between the ages of 10 and 15; in nearly a quarter of obsessional neurotics the condition has become established by the age of 15; and by the age of 30 nearly three quarters of the cases. The development of the illness is usually insidious with about 7 years between onset and psychiatric referral. Precipitating factors held responsible have included illness and injury, conflict especially marital difficulties, and important life passages, such as the menarche, marriage, pregnancy and child birth, and also the experience of loss in bereavement. It is the patient's perception of these events which is important in provoking symptoms. Times of stress are often associated with an exacerbation of symptoms, and so the natural history appears episodic. Disorder of mood may also precipitate obsessional symptoms in the predisposed. In some patients symptoms remain severe with little diminution over very many years.

Good prognosticators include: an episodic nature of the illness; presence of external precipitating factors; disorder of mood; short duration of illness with onset in early adult life. Obsessions starting in childhood and occurring continuously or repetitively through adolescence, carry a worse prognosis; as does single marital status. It has been claimed that obsessional symptoms give some protection from suicide; however, the rate for suicide is higher than in the healthy population. At follow-up obsessional patients are very rarely found to have been rediagnosed schizophrenia. Although the obsessional rumination involves thinking about acts which are repulsive to the patient and grossly socially unacceptable, obscene or criminal, in fact it is very uncommon for these thoughts to be acted upon, and it is reasonable to reassure patients absolutely about their fears of acting out obsessional ruminations.

A man of 37 described a steady increase of obsessional symptoms over 12 years. He worked as an engineer but was quite unable to function because every time he had to count numbers he would need to check his figures more than twenty times. He had elaborate rituals involving getting into lifts, walking alongside another person and even getting in and out of his car that would require a great deal of checking and touching. Sometimes it would take him 45 minutes to leave his car after arriving in the car park. He became increasingly miserable and despondent about his inability to cope with life.

Some degree of anxiety and reactive depression is often associated with obsessional neurosis. The irresistible nature of the obsession, and the limitation this places on the patient's social life cause understandable misery. Occasionally this secondary depression may become very severe and require treatment. Not infrequently it is the depressive symptoms that are primary and the patient has reacted to these with obsessional symptoms.

Neurotic Depression

Neurotic depression is the commonest of neurotic syndromes, but poorly defined. A few of the many meanings of the term 'depression', as used in the International Classification, are shown in figure 6.4. The origins of the concept 'melancholia' and the classical argument as to whether depressive illness is unitary or two different conditions has been well summarised by Snaith (1981). Endogenous or psychotic

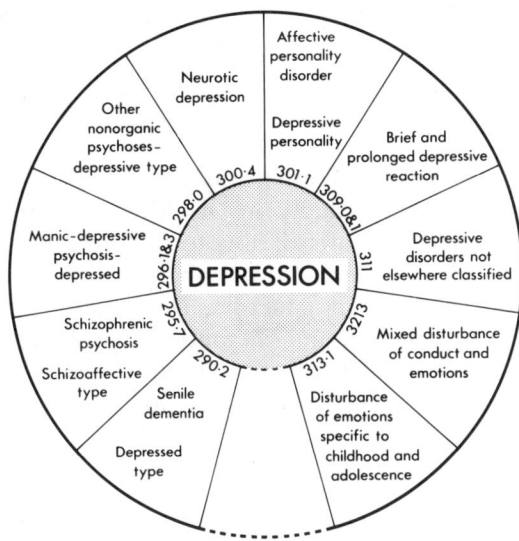

Figure 6.4   Ten uses of the term 'Depression'

depression is a reasonably definite nosological entity, but neurotic depression is not nearly so clearcut.

It is common to find that there are features of both endogenous and neurotic depression present. From the point of view of practical management, it is best to diagnose in two stages. First, is endogenous depression present? If so, this should be appropriately treated. Second, to what extent is neurosis causing distress and failure to cope? If to any considerable extent, then treatment for neurosis should be carried out. There is often a neurotic reaction following the successful treatment of clearcut endogenous depression.

It is difficult to decide whether symptoms are those of neurosis or affective psychosis; depressive 'state' as neurotic depression, or depressive 'trait' in dysthymic personality disorder; depressive neurosis with anxiety, anxiety neurosis with depression, or both. It is often difficult to separate the understandable states of unhappiness associated with the acute reaction to stress and grief from neurotic depression. However, in a neurotic condition depression is disproportionate to the distressing experiences. There is usually preoccupation with the precipitating psychological event. The depression is inappropriate, that is continuing after the provoking circumstances have been removed, and impairing the patient's ability to cope with circumstances. Neurotic or reactive depression has sometimes been called 'situational depression' to distinguish it from endogenous depression where no external precipitant is expected. However, Hirschfield (1981) has cast doubt on separation between two syndromes according to presence of external cause; he found an equal amount of external stress in both types of depression and equal disturbance of personality, but symptomatic differences were found between the two groups. Those patients with situational depression showed more overt anger and self-pity.

Neurotic depression characteristically has a fairly sudden onset in response to a precipitant usually in the form of a provoking stress ascribed by the patient and identifiable to the observer. The intensity of symptoms varies at different times and responds to exacerbating and ameliorating (neutralising) factors. Depression is usually worse in the afternoon or evening, and the patient has difficulty in getting off to sleep. Other neurotic features or abnormality of personality may be in evidence with self-pity and hypochondriacal ideas, irritability and general difficulty in coping, in addition to misery. There may also be hysterical or obsessional features.

The association between depression and socio-economic conditions within the city was investigated in Plymouth (Dean and James, 1980). A high rate for neurotic depression in males was associated with various social factors. Wards of the city with the highest male re-admission rate for depressive neurosis were those with above average rates for households in council accommodation, above average rented unfurnished accommodation, and below average number of households with all basic amenities; and also above average of retired persons and one person households. The association was less marked for females with depressive neurosis. There is there-fore some positive correlation between frequency of depressive neurosis and poorer socio-economic conditions.

The overwhelming majority of mental disorders seen in general practice are neurotic, and most of these depressive. So the population characteristics of depressive neurosis are similar to neuroses in general. It most commonly occurs following misfortunes, especially losses, and with feelings of loss of self esteem. Depressive neurosis is more likely to occur where there is premorbid disorder of personality.

In Brown and Harris' (1978) studies of women in an urban population survey, 17% were suffering from recognisable psychiatric syndromes, almost entirely affective in nature, mostly neurotic depression. Another source of epidemiological data, as mentioned in chapter 3, is the Second National Study of Morbidity Statistics from General Practice (O.P.C.S., 1974). The morbidity and diagnoses of more than 290,000 patients all over England and Wales was recorded by more than 100 general practitioners in 1971-72. The rates per 1000 patients consulting in general practice were as fol-lows: for all mental disorders 109.9; for affective psychoses 4.1 and for depressive neurosis 31.4. Thus family doctors reckoned that there were nearly eight times as many suffering from neurotic depression as from endogenous depression amongst surgery attenders.

Psychotic or endogenous depression is a discrete condition and probably has a genetic or biochemical basis, while neurotic depression, so-called, is not a single condition, but describes many different ways in which the patient tries to cope with his own neuroticism and perceived stress (Kiloh *et al.*, 1972). Thus depressive psychosis would seem to be 'a disease', but neurotic depression more a manifestation of a general neurotic condition that merges in its presentation and natural history with other neuroses.

We will now discuss some of the aetiological theories that have been used to explain neurotic depression. The model of the affect of hopelessness is useful in portraying the origins of neurotic depression described in chapter 4. There is considered to be an association between the presence of this affect and serious physical illness. Engel considers that it 'contributes to the emergence of somatic disease . . . if the necessary predisposing factors are present . . . . When man gives up psychologically he disrupts the continuity of his relatedness to himself and his many environments . . . with this loss of continuity he may become more vulnerable to pathogenic influences. These would constitute failures or complications of the *flight-fight* or *conservation-withdrawal* systems as biological defences'.

The giving-up given-up complex (Engel, 1968) evokes the psychodynamic concept of depression — object loss. Parkes (1972) has demonstrated the similarities in emotional response to different kinds of loss — a home, a limb, a spouse. The numbness which is the initial response to the experience of loss is followed by panic and searching behaviour which may be quite extreme and bizarre on occasions. Searching is exemplified by the pseudo-hallucinations for the presence of the dead person in bereavement, or by the morbid thoughts of the amputee as to 'what have they done with my leg?'. The next stage of realisation of loss is associated with grieving and reactive depression.

Depression is linked with loss of self-esteem. Guilty feelings are, of course, a prominent symptom in depression, that is depression causes feelings of loss of self-esteem; it is also caused by it. A happening of which a person is very ashamed is often the trigger for depressive illness. Significantly, loss of self-esteem is an important contributor to the suffering caused by the loss of a 'loved object'. The widow feels acutely the loss of status occasioned by her bereavement; the amputee feels mutilated and less able to face the world.

'Introjection' has been suggested as a mechanism for depression. A person of rigid personality self-controlled in the extreme, is unable to express his strong antipathy for others. In conflict, he turns these feelings of aggression in on himself with resultant self-blame and depression. In Gestalt psychology, a person finds his position in and attitude towards the world meaningless, and the resultant emptiness is experienced as depression.

One of the many different behavioural formulations for the origins of depression is as follows. Life involves ceaseless activity of seeking and responding to reinforcers both obvious and subtle, immediate and more remote. The abnormality in depression can be seen to be loss of reinforcement. There is of course much argument as to whether this is due to object loss, social reinforcement, loss of patient's reinforceable behaviour, loss of the effectiveness of the reinforcers, or aversive behaviour preventing the possibility of receiving reinforcement. In clinical practice all these occur in de-pression but it seems to be an explanation of the behaviour result-ing from neurotic depression rather than demonstration of cause.

Seligman's behavioural model of learned helplessness (1975) based on animal experiments has also been discussed in chapter 4. Depression, in this model, is the belief in one's own helplessness. The patient comes to accept that there is nothing he can do to avoid the adversities of life.

It must be reiterated that neurotic depression is not sharply de-marcated from other sorts of neurosis. Although the mood is con-spicuously impaired, all other areas of thinking and experiencing are disturbed as well. This was expressed in a poem entitled 'Purgatory at All Saints Hospital' by a patient, who wrote:

> 'My God, my God where do I belong?
> Let not your heart be troubled. Sylvia said
> The trouble enters not only the heart but
> also the head.'

Neurasthenia

This is a neurotic reaction characterised by lack of psychological and physical energy. The symptoms are lassitude, difficulty in concentration, fatigue, disturbed sleep, headache, irritability and lack of capacity for enjoyment. Such patients present more often in general practice than in the psychiatric clinic, as these symptoms are usually transient. A distinction is made between neurasthenia as a neurotic reaction and the asthenic personality disorder. Neuras-thenia is commoner with asthenic personality disorder, and the two overlap to a considerable extent. Neurasthenia is often associated with psychogenic stress, especially the acute external stress such as occurs in a major disaster, and after physical illness, of which virus conditions such as influenza, glandular fever or infective hepatitis are especially notorious. The mood of listlessness, apathy and anergia may progress into overt depression. Neurasthenia is an old fashioned and unfashionable diagnosis, but it still retains usefulness for patients with these limited symptoms.

Age of onset and mode of presentation is very variable. Neurasthenia is particularly likely in a busy person, who fails to make as rapid and full a recovery after a physical illness or severe emotional stress as would be expected under the circumstances. It may also occur quite commonly in the recovery stage from a psychotic illness, for example, following depression or schizophrenia. This is probably not part of the major illness itself, but much more a neurotic reaction to the failure to cope, loss of self-esteem and anxiety over social status that having suffered such an illness engenders. It is especially noticeable in the recovery phase of professional people following a major depressive illness.

A clerk who had prided himself on his good work record and physical fitness had a severe acute depressive illness. He made a complete recovery. Exactly a year later he presented with feelings of listlessness, irritability and generalised physical symptoms. He described himself as 'less than 100%' and clearly had suffered a massive loss of confidence following his illness although he was not now clinically depressed.

A situation in which one needs to be wary if the diagnosis neurasthenia is used is the post-concussional syndrome (Taylor, 1967). The symptomatology of this syndrome after head injury is very similar to the classical description of neurasthenia. There is a higher rate of so-called neuroticism after head trauma. However the evidence that this is truly neurotic is not convincing; there is often intellectual as well as emotional impairment and diffuse minor organic lesions remain a possibility.

Depersonalisation Syndrome

Depersonalisation has already been described earlier in this chapter, as the unpleasant perception of the person's own body or external objects (derealisation) experienced as being altered in quality, unreal or distant. Depersonalisation may occur in isolation in neurotic patients but its frequent occurrence with severe anxiety and phobic symptoms has been incorporated by Roth (1959) within the 'phobic anxiety depersonalisation syndrome'. Like other phobic disorders, this is most frequently seen in younger married women. On detailed enquiry, some depersonalisation symptoms are elicited from the majority of neurotic sufferers.

Hypochondriasis

Hypochondriasis is a preoccupation with symptoms or illness. It is best considered not as the name of a disease, but as an adjective; hypochondriacal neurosis may manifest as: fears about the development of physical or mental illness without any associated symptoms; belief that actual symptoms are of dire and serious consequence; or, experience of normal bodily sensation of consciousness as unpleasant symptoms. Hypochondriasis is a disorder of the content of mental experience, and not necessarily neurotic in origin. It may occur with depressive psychosis or associated with somatic symptoms in schizophrenia. It may also occur with other neuroses. Chronic hypochondriacal neurosis is both common and extremely intractable.

Hypochondriacal neurosis occurs in both sexes. Its onset is likely to be associated with precipitating factors, especially those life events that have physical sequelae, such as a coronary thrombosis in an athletic man. The involutional period in both sexes is a particularly likely time for the onset of hypochondriacal symptoms. A woman may have fears of her loss of sexual attractiveness; a man is more likely to be concerned with loss of virility and physical fitness. Hypochondriasis occurs also during pregnancy and in the puerperium, and is commonly seen in adolescence in both sexes. It is more conspicuous in those groups of people who for occupational or other reasons demand of themselves peak physical performance at all times.

Hypochondriacal symptoms most commonly occur in the musculo-skeletal system with various aches, pains and limitation of function, the gastro-intestinal system with indigestion, constipation and preoccupation with bowel function, and the central nervous system, especially headache (Kenyon, 1976). The head and neck, abdomen and chest are commonly affected but almost any other part of the body may be also. In 16% of cases symptoms were predominantly unilateral, and of these 73% left-sided. Of patients admitted with a diagnosis of hypochondriasis, 47% showed no physical abnormality; in 70% pain was a prominent symptom. Hypochondriasis may occur for mental as well as bodily symptoms, for example, in those patients who are preoccupied with a fear of going mad.

Attention has been paid to psychogenic bodily complaints in chapter 3, and so these are not dealt with further at this stage. It is important to note that patients may express with their bodies emotions that they seem unable to convey in words. This inability to express emotion verbally has been called 'alexithymia'.

The Manifestation of Symptoms

Like other people, the neurotic strives for internal consistency. He works at demonstrating to himself and to others that he and the world he lives in are really as he claims them to be. He feels it is impossible to cope, that all possible ways of dealing with present problems will be ultimately futile. Although there is no defect of perception, he is highly selective in how perception is interpreted so that this validates his views of his own world. The way he sees all outside circumstances are skewed. He comes to ignore all evidence that would contradict this opinion, and this increases the intractableness of the condition. Eventually he reaches the situation where illness is the only logical and acceptable state in which he can remain.

The 'internal restlessness' (Vere, 1778), of neurosis is manifested in emotion — that is in depression or misery, anxiety or fear. The internal emotional state may be converted into behaviour — hysterical conversion or disassociation, or illness behaviour. Thinking is distracted in achieving its goals by neurotic misinterpretation of relationships or by obsessional ideas. The expression of neurotic symptomatology is very different but the impairment of functioning is shared to a greater or lesser extent.

Hysteria, anxiety, hypochondriasis should not be thought of as entirely separate conditions but rather as adjectival descriptions of the type of neurosis. What sort of neurosis is it? Is it an hysterical or hypochondriacal neurosis, or a neurosis with features of anxiety, phobia and depersonalisation.

Bibliography

Barker, J.C. (1962). The syndrome of hospital addiction (Munchausen's syndrome). *J. ment. Sci.*, 108, 167–182

Beech, H.R. (1974). *Obsessional States*, Methuen, London

Brown, G.W. and Harris, T. (1978). *Social Origins of Depression*, Tavistock Publications, London

Chodoff, P. and Lyons, H. (1958). Hysteria, the hysterical personality and hysterical conversion. *Am. J. Psychiat.*, 114, 734–40

Dean, K.G. and James, H.D. (1980). The spatial distribution of depressive illness in Plymouth. *Br. J. Psychiat.*, 136, 167–80

Dostoievski, F.M. (1846). *The Double*, Penguin Books, Harmondsworth

Engel, G.L. (1968). A life setting conducive to illness. The giving-up given-up complex. *Ann. int. Med.*, 69, 293–300

Ganser, S.J. (1898). Veber einen eigenartigan hysterischen Daminszustand. *Archiv Psychiatrie Nervenkrankheiten*, 30, 633–640. Trans. Shorer, C.E., 1965, *Br. J. Crimin.*, 5, 120–126

Hay, G.G. (1970). Psychiatric aspects of cosmetic nasal operations. *Br. J. Psychiat.*, 115, 85–97

Hirschfield, R.M.A. (1981). Situational depression: Validity of the concept. *Br. J. Psychiat.*, 139, 297-305

Jaspers, K. (1962). *General Psychopathology*, translated from German 7th Ed. by Hoenig, J. and Hamilton, M.W., University Press, Manchester

Jovanovic, U.J. (1978). Sleep profile and ultradian sleep periodicity in neurotic patients compared with the corresponding parameters in healthy human subjects. *Waking & Sleeping*, 2, 47-55

Kenyon, F.E. (1976). Hypochondriacal states. *Br. J. Psychiat.*, 129, 1-14

Kiloh, L.G., Andrews, G., Neilson, M. and Bianchi, G.N. (1972). The relationship of the syndromes called exogenus and neurotic depression. *Br. J. Psychiat.*, 121, 183-196

Leff, J.P. (1978). Psychiatrists' versus Patients' concepts of unpleasant emotions. *Br. J. Psychiat.*, 133, 306-13

Lewis, A.J. (1975). The survival of hysteria. *Psychol. Med.*, 5, 9-12

Lewis, C. Day (1948). The Neurotic. *Poems 1943-1947*

Marks, I.M. (1970). The classification of phobia disorders. *Br. J. Psychiat.*, 116, 377-386

Marks, I.M. (1981). Space 'phobia': a pseudo-agoraphobic syndrome. *J. Neurol., Neurosurg. Psychiat.*, 44, 387-391

Mechanic, D. (1966). Response factors in illness: The study of illness behaviour. *Soc. Psychiat.*, 1, 11-20

Merskey, H. (1979). *The Analysis of Hysteria*, Baillière Tindall, London

Office of Population Censuses and Surveys (1974). *Morbidity Statistics for General Practice: Second National Study* 1970-71, H.M.S.O., London

Parkes, C.M. (1972). Components of the reaction to loss of a limb, spouse or home. *J. Psychosom. Res.*, 16, 343

Perley, M.J. and Guze, S.B. (1962). Hysteria - the stability and usefulness of clinical criteria. A quantitative study based on a follow-up period of 6-8 years in 39 patients. *New Eng. J. Med.*, 266, 421-426

Prince, M. (1905). *The Dissociation of a Personality*, Longmans, New York

Roth, M. (1959). The phobic anxiety depersonalization syndrome. *Proc. R. Soc. Med.*, 52, 587-596

Seligman, M.E.P. (1975). *Helplessness*, San Francisco, Freeman

Slater, E. (1965). Diagnosis of hysteria. *Br. med. J.*, 1, 1395-9

Slater, E. and Roth, M. (1969). *Clinical Psychiatry*, 3rd edn, Baillière Tindall, London

Snaith, R.P. (1981). *Clinical Neurosis*, Oxford University Press

Stevenson, R.L. (1925). *Dr. Jekyll and Mr. Hyde*, Dent, London and Toronto

Taylor, A.R. (1967). Post concussional sequelae. *Br. med. J.*, 2, 67-71

Tonks, C.M. (1975). Premenstrual tension. In: *Contemporary Psychiatry* (Ed. Silverstone, T. and Barraclough, B.), Headly Brothers, Ashford, Kent

Trimble, M.R. (1981). *Post-traumatic Neurosis*, John Wiley, Chichester

Vere, James (1778). A physical and moral enquiry into the causes of that internal restlessness and disorder in man, which has been the complaint of all ages, London White & Sewell, cited by Hunter & MacAlpine

W.H.O. (1977). *Manual of the International Classification of Diseases*, 9th Revision, W.H.O., Geneva

7 Neurosis and Personality Disorder

'Can the Ethiopian change his skin; or the leopard his spots?'
Jeremiah 13:23

Neurotic behaviour implies carrying out an act in response to a stressor in a manner that is inappropriate to deal with that stress; for example, the husband who breaks down his own front door with his fists because his wife locks him out. Neurotic illness is a consistent pattern of maladaptive behaviour occurring over a longer time in response to either a prolonged stress, or a stress with long term repercussions; for example, the young woman who cannot, because of chronic anxiety, separate from her mother and so spends her time at her family home rather than with her husband, so jeopardising her marriage. 'Neurotic personality', 'neuroticism', 'abnormality of personality' or 'personality disorder' is a life-long characteristic in the context of which such reactions of behaviour or illness may occur; for example, the exessively cautious sensitive schoolboy chooses his future occupation partly because of his personality constitution, and becomes the over-conscientious, fussy bank clerk constantly worried by scruples of detail. He is more prone to anxiety neurosis of his personality structure.

Personality theory, and especially the clinical list of the International Classification (World Health Organization, 1977) seems untidy and unscientific. Nevertheless it does have some value. Accurate observation and categorisation of personality can be useful practically because it is predictive. You can expect with a reasonable degree of certainty that your patient with an obsessive, meticulous personality will respond to circumstances, for example learning to live as a diabetic on insulin, in one way whilst a histrionic person will react quite differently.

What is Personality Disorder?

Personality and personality disorder are abstract concepts and yet enormously influential on the person's whole life. One cannot in any comprehensive way measure personality; what is important clinically is different from the parameters described by research psychologists. Many different definitions with overlapping meanings confuse the issue in personality and personality disorder. However, there are two main senses in which the term is used clinically. First, it is taken to mean all those problems arising from abnormality of the personality, whether they affect the person himself or those around him. The second sense refers specifically to those problems associated with asocial personality disorder; that is, the term conveys social disapproval. In this chapter we will take the first, more comprehensive definition, although we will refer to asocial personality disorder as one type. How the clinical notion of 'personality disorder' is derived from evaluation of personality is summarised in table 7.1. There has been a vast amount written about personality; the reader wishing to be familiarised with this should consult a basic textbook of psychology; in this chapter there is only space to discuss the psychiatric concept of personality disorder.

The definition of personality disorder in the 9th Revision of The International Classification of Diseases reads, 'deeply ingrained maladaptive patterns of behaviour generally recognisable by the time of adolescence or earlier and continuing throughout most of adult life, although often becoming less obvious in middle or old age. The personality is abnormal either in the balance of its components, their quality and expression or in its total aspect. Because of this deviation or psychopathy the patient suffers or others have to suffer and there is an adverse effect upon the individual or on society'. So this definition takes the broader view of personality disorder, but includes within it the narrower aspect of asocial personality disorder or psychopathy.

Table 7.1   Building up a profile of personality disorder

What is meant by personality?

    Subjective: aims and goals
    Objective: consistent pattern of behaviour

Is the personality normal or abnormal?

    Statistical variation from the norm

What abnormal characteristics are clinically important?

    Typological lists as in table 7.2

What abnormalities of personality amount to disorder?

    Where this causes the person himself
    or others to suffer

Personality is one of those vexing topics in life which we know something about and yet have great difficulty in defining. Subjectively, personality 'is the unique quality of the individual his feelings and personal goals' (Schneider, 1958). Objectively, personality may be considered as the characteristic pattern of behaviour of an individual; what makes him different from other people; the way we can predict that he will act in any particular circumstances. Personality includes his prevailing mood, thinking and attitudes, but excludes intelligence and physical constitution. It is manifested in social relationships, 'and can be regarded as consisting of what people actually do in social contexts. To diagnose personality the clinician is called upon to explore by clinical interview, the person's pattern of relationships with other people (including his behaviour to the clinician himself)' (Walton and Presly, 1973).

When we talk about normality of personality we should use the term 'normal' in its scientific sense, that is the statistical norm. For example, an Englishman 5'8" tall is normal; to be 6'2" or 5'2" tall is equally abnormal. Consigning the height of such people to the category of 'abnormality' is not a value judgment, nor does it comment on whether they are taller or shorter than normal. Normality and abnormality of personality should be assessed in the same way. Abnormal personality is a variation upon an accepted yet broadly conceived range of average personality; that is, it is statistically abnormal. The variation may be expressed as an excess or a deficiency of certain qualities of the personality. Thus, it is not a value judgment to say that the personality is abnormal. The person may have much more of a desired personality characteristic than normal; St. Francis of Assisi might be regarded as having been abnormal in personality because he showed much more of the characteristics of charity and kindness towards his fellows than normal. Much less of these qualities than normal may be manifested by a callous tyrant who is therefore also regarded as abnormal. In terms of normality or abnormality both people are equally abnormal, but their abnormality is not in the same direction.

This way of assessing personality according to types considers that the characteristics of these types conform to a normal distribution; a person of normal personality has the quality (like charitableness) to a normal extent; it is abnormal to have much more or much less of this characteristic. Schneider's personality types were assumed to be normally distributed in this way. Essen-Möller (1956) carried out a clinical survey of personality of 2250 people living in a rural community in Sweden. He assessed personality characteristics, and later Sjobring (1973) developed these ideas about the clinical nature of personality in which he considered three dimensions of personality

occurred with normal distribution curves. These he called *stability*,
solidity and *validity*. Eysencks' (1969) description of *extraversion*
has close similarities to Sjobring's *substable*. Eysenck described *extraversion* and *introversion* as lying on one axis, and *neuroticism* and
stability on another at 90 degrees. This description of personality by
Eysenck has had extensive use in research but is less relevant in
clinical medicine.

Certain aspects of personality are found to be clinically important,
including relationships with other people, whether the subject believes
that control for his course of action lies within himself or with others,
self-estimation, consistent level of mood and energy, moral and
ethical standards, interests and habits, and typical reactions to stress.
These aspects have traditionally been collected into lists, for example
that of Schneider in which personality types were considered to
occur with a normal distribution; the International Classification of
Diseases category of personality disorder (I.C.D. 9: 301) has been
derived from this.

Using cluster analysis, Tyrer and Alexander (1979) found five
discrete categories in the abnormal personality of psychiatric patients.
They consider that the current classification of personality could be
simplified using these criteria. These three typological classifications

Table 7.2   Typological classification of personality disorder

Schneider, 1958	International Classification, 1977	Tyrer and Alexander, 1979
Hyperthymic	Affective	Dysthymic
Depressive	Schizoid	Schizoid
Insecure Sensitive Anankastic	Anankastic	Anankastic
Attention-seeking	Hysterical	Passive dependence
Labile		
Asthenic	Asthenic	
Fanatic	Paranoid	Sociopathy
Explosive	Explosive	
Affectionless	Asocial	
Weak-willed		

of personality disorder (Schneider, I.C.D. and Tyrer) are compared in table 7.2. Personality disorder is present when the abnormality of personality causes the person himself to suffer, or other people to suffer. The social environment is all important in dictating whether personality disorder manifests or not. A misfit in one station of life may well be a success in another. The socially unacceptable psychopath of one society could well have been a charismatic patriotic leader in another social setting; Genghis Khan for example, might well have proved an uncomfortable fellow-citizen in a modern European metropolis. This means that whether abnormal personality is regarded as disorder or not depends, in part, on social circumstances; it is not an absolute diagnosis but a threshold phenomenon and social circumstances alter the threshold. In clinical practice it has been found that personality disorders differ only in degree from the personalities of other psychiatric patients.

Development of Personality

The derivation of our ideas on personality and its development have been traced in chapter 2. The seeds of abnormality in adult life are looked for in inheritance and childhood development. When London's water supply was in danger during the drought of 1976, the upper reaches of the Thames were examined more critically. Similarly in understanding disturbed behaviour arising from personality disorder, it is worth considering how that personality developed. The personality of adults, the patterns which mould their behaviour, are relatively fixed. There is a slight degree of change in response to the environment, but inflexibility is more conspicuous. The cautious, rigid, conscientious person tends to stay that way in whatever circumstances he finds himself, and these characteristics continue from childhood onwards.

There has been discussion in chapter 4 concerning the relative importance of heredity and environment in the development of personality. This is in many ways a sterile wrangle as the two cannot be separated. Both genetics and early experience mould the way a person reacts. The true complexity of the situation is to some extent revealed by the use of the same word for different types of acquisition. We may inherit blue eyes from our father (genetic); we may also inherit the capacity for running a business (genetic and early upbringing); we may also inherit the business itself (environmental). The environmental influences on a person could be said to include both the sort of home they are brought up in and also the conditions in the uterus of their mother before birth, for example placental insufficiency. So the arguments between heredity and environment become tortuous and tautologous.

Types of Personality Disorder

The characteristics of the personality types listed below occur in people without disorder; but when they result in major disadvantage to the person himself or to those around him, this is personality disorder. The following types are those whose use is recommended by the International Classification. It is far from ideal as a classification, but it has the advantage of wide use.

Paranoid Personality Disorder

The distinctive feature of this type of personality is self-reference; that is, these are people who misinterpret the words and actions of others as having special significance for, and being directed against themselves. They misconstrue other people, they are suspicious, they feel that others are unduly aware of them, and taking notice of them in an antagonistic and derogatory way. There are two main subgroups of this personality type and these will be described separately.

The active type of paranoid personality disorder is a suspicious person with an aggressive and unaccepting manner. He is quarrelsome, litiginous, often going to elaborate lengths to defend his rights, and to redress real or imagined injustices. He is intensely jealous of what he regards as his own belongings, whether these are objects or people, and he spends a lot of time talking about and planning to 'get his own back'. He is often seen as self-important and fanatical. This is the sort of person who, seeing a footpath marked on his map across a field as a right of way, will march resolutely across the field of growing wheat despite the irate farmer with a shotgun at the far side. He provides the lawyers with business and may be a useful catalyst in the community, but he can also be very destructive within the closer human exchanges of the family.

The passive type of paranoid personality faces the world from a position of submission and humiliation. He assumes that whatever happens to him will be done for the worst. He is just as suspicious and self-referrent as the active type, and misconstrues circumstances and other people. He feels that his friends are likely to let him down, and when he meets new people he assumes that they will either dislike him or ignore him.

Such people retain their characteristics of personality life long. In old age they may be cantankerous, hostile activists or morose, suspicious, vulnerable misanthropists. Because of the way they see relationships they tend to create difficulties for themselves, and so their fears and feelings of self-reference are often self-fulfilling.

Affective Personality Disorder

Again, there are two main types of affective personality disorder. The first are those whose mood is persistently anxious, gloomy or depressive. Their attitude to life is either one of prevailing depression and misery, or of vague but uncomfortable anxiety. The mood is pronounced and life long. It is therefore a depressive or anxious *trait*, and not an evanescent *state* of depression or anxiety. Such persistently dysthymic people are often gentle and likeable, but their whole approach to life is tinged with gloom or apprehensiveness. Everything is seen through purple tinted spectacles, 'every silver lining has a cloud'. 'There are no circumstances in life that are so bad as to be incapable of further deterioration.'

The other main type of affective personality disorder is the cyclothymic personality. Such people show very marked fluctuations of mood. For a day, or a week, they may be optimistic, energetic, garrulous, full of ideas and plans; then the next week they become gloomy, morose and taciturn. Such cycles may be linked to other biological rhythms, for example the menstrual cycle, but may be independent of this, irregular and unpredictable. Cyclothymic personality does to some extent predispose to frank affective disorder, and has on occasions been treated successfully by measures normally reserved for treating mood disorders.

There are a few people who have persistently elated mood as a feature of their personality. However such a person is unlikely to be referred for psychiatric treatment. He does not himself suffer, although he may on occasion cause social embarrassment.

Schizoid Personality Disorder

There is considerable argument whether this personality is associated with greater frequency of developing schizophrenic illness or not. In fact the association appears to be tenuous. Such personalities are characterised by withdrawal from social involvement, and emotional coolness and detachment.

They show a disinclination to mix with other people, appearing somewhat aloof. They lack interest in the company of others but their mood is not depressed, and their separation from human society is not due to shyness or sensitivity. They are solitary and appear lonely, but in fact prefer not to be involved in social occupations. Their interests and hobbies usually tend to increase their isolation from other people.

Those closely related to them may complain of their emotional detachment, their inability to inspire strong feelings in others, and their callous indifference towards other people. They tend to be interested rather than involved, concerned with things rather than people. A group of 20 young men who had been former child psychiatric patients and diagnosed as having schizoid personality were compared with a control group at follow-up (Chick *et al.*, 1979). The former schizoid subjects were found to use psychological constructs less than the control group. This was assessed by asking subjects to comment on the differences between people in pairs of photographs. Various categories of difference were commented upon (occupation, activity, clothes, etc.), but only comments about psychological characteristics differed significantly between the two groups of subjects; these findings suggested a deficit amongst the schizoid individuals which may be related specifically to their lack of empathy. It would suggest that the schizoid features in childhood remain into young adult life.

Explosive Personality Disorder

The main characteristic of these people is liability to intemperate outbursts of mood. With apparently slight provocation they become angry or irritable, even potentially violent. They are treated with circumspection by other people who know them well, with 'kid gloves'; because of this they tend to get their own way due to their ill humour. They may exploit other people's fears of them to gain their own ends. Such personalities tend to be unpopular and disruptive. Fortunately they are only met with uncommonly.

Such people behave normally for most of the time and only occasionally explode in impulsive irritability. Because of their ability to establish normal relationships at other times they do get involved with others and their outbursts then tend to give them a dominant role in a relationship, for example the arbitrarily aggressive, violent husband whose wife is completely dominated by him.

Anankastic Personality Disorder

Anankastic or obsessional personality occurs frequently. Such a person has many assets that make him a valuable member of society. There are two main groups of features in this personality type which overlap to a considerable extent; feelings of insecurity and meticulous conscientiousness. The pervading sense of insecurity is associated with great self-doubt and feelings of sensitivity concerning how other people view him. He may be shy, awkward in company and have difficulty expressing his strongly felt emotion.

The meticulous conscientiousness shows itself in perfectionism and rigidity. He carries out his duties at work with precision and attention to detail. He may often be tidy, houseproud to a fault; 'I must put my pyjamas in the drawer marked pyjamas' (Dylan Thomas). He is very upset by the slightest suspicion of criticism and 'takes it very much to heart'. The importance he attaches to others' opinions of himself makes him a conformist; rigid and formal in his social and moral attitudes or behaviour.

Insecurity about his ability and his relationships makes the anankast indecisive. He doubts his own capacity and only too easily finds himself secretly agreeing with those who criticise him. He vacillates and has great difficulty in making choices. Insight into the limitation of his personality may cause him to over-compensate, which he will do with his characteristic obsessional thoroughness. He may then deliberately make decisions arbitrarily upon insufficient evidence, deliberately be untidy, or compensate for his legalistic rigidity by flaunting the law intentionally. His basic obsessionality however is still manifest. With his doubts and vacillations he has a considerable capacity for looking at situations from different points of view. This ability results in an attitude of ambivalence, continually weighing up the pros and cons. He finds the initiation or completion of any activity difficult, but he will slave away at the part of the job in the middle indefinitely .

The discipline and conscientiousness of the obsessional make him a useful person in an organisation but he is difficult to live with. As he ages he becomes more rigid and intolerant, with his attitudes from a previous generation causing friction with his younger relatives brought up with different mores. His chronic indecisiveness becomes more pronounced with the ageing process and also if there is superimposed brain damage. This may make life difficult for those around him. The tendency to criticise himself may make him miserable. There is an increased likelihood for such people to develop depression.

He values accuracy and thoroughness highly and respects other obsessionals for their quality of obsessionality. He is always extremely aware of what other people are thinking about him and he feels that consistency to the extent of being inflexible is expected of him. He shows extreme self-control and readily finds fault in himself. Some of these characteristics are extremely common in the general population and it is only when they are present to a very marked extent, and when they cause suffering to the person himself or to those around him that anankastic personality disorder is present.

Hysterical Personality Disorder

This is quite different from hysterical neurosis and it is unfortunate that the same adjective qualifies both. It occurs in females more often than males. Perhaps 'histrionic' would be a better description for the personality type, because, the word has a different derivation from hysterical, and is aptly descriptive of the characteristic behaviour. The use of the term hysterical is highly confused and unstandardised. De Alarcon (1973) summarised the description 22 authors gave for hysterical personality and found that they had listed 28 different traits of personality. Greatest agreement by the 14 authors who gave 6 or more characteristics was upon histrionic behaviour (85% of authors), egocentricity (78%), emotional lability (70%), excitability (70%), dependency (70%), suggestibility (57%), and seductiveness (57%).

A fundamental characteristic of the hysterical personality is the shallowness and lability of emotion that they demonstrate. They form excellent and rapid superficial relationships with new people, but they have great difficulty sustaining a close, long term, mutually rewarding, exclusive relationship. Mood is fluctuating and inconsistent and extreme attention-, affection-, and appreciation-craving from others is shown. Such a person may be histrionic and over-dramatic, and her excessive involvement with many different people in a short space of time is seen as manipulativeness. There is often a degree of theatricality about the way situations in human relationships are set up. This personality has at times been considered a female equivalent of the asocial or psychopathic personality, which is commoner in men. In a study of hospital patients considered to have hysterical personality disorder, Thompson (1980) found 83% of subjects to be female. There was a clear association with neurotic depression; 73% gave a history of overdosage and 27% of self-mutilation. Addiction, especially to alcohol, occurred in half of these patients; a history of violence and criminality was common.

Immaturity in sexual relationships is a common feature of the hysterical personality. Characteristically such people make initial flirtatious advances and then recoil into frigidity when the liaison threatens to become more meaningful. This stance in sexual behaviour, beckoning and then rejecting results in frustrated, fractured relationships. In family matters, the hysterical personality often retains control and dominance but at the same time creates distress and distrust. She is charming and sociable but at the same time inconsistent, and creates disharmony amongst those around her. She makes demands for love and attention which she cannot match from her own limited emotional resources. The long lasting relationships of such people, for example, their marriages, tend to go wrong. Hysterical personalities demonstrate a need for change and excitement. They are at the same time excessively dependent upon other people, making great emotional demands upon them, and also controlling. Their manipulation of others often fails to achieve useful objectives and may eventually prove destructive.

Asthenic Personality Disorder

The asthenic personality conforms most closely to that common epithet, the 'inadequate personality'. The person is lacking in mental energy and the ability to react to changing demands. He lacks confidence to cope with problems. He may function reasonably well and appear quite inconspicuous when carried along through life by a dominant close relationship. However when external stress occurs, he copes poorly and may break down. He craves long term support and encouragement from relatives, the general practitioner, social worker, minister, employer or surrounding social organisation. For example, he may survive very well in the Services but be completely unable to adjust to unstructured civilian life.

Characteristically, such a person is dependent upon his parents, especially his mother. He may, partly at his mother's instigation, marry the girl next door who then takes over his mother's role. Crises may be precipitated by the marriage breaking down, or by losing his job, or after physical illness; and it is following such crises that he may come to the attention of the helping professions. Dependence amounts to passive compliance with the aims and demands of the more dominant partner. There is a lack of vigour in holding aims and goals, and in all he attempts to carry out.

Asocial Personality Disorder

In the asocial personality (antisocial or psychopathic personality) the defect is primarily one of empathy; the ability to understand other people's feelings, and especially to understand how other people feel about the consequences of the person's own actions. A normal person is prevented most of the time by shame or psychological pain from carrying out unpleasant actions towards somebody else. He does not want to be disliked and feels very keenly what it would be like to be at the receiving end of such behaviour. It is this ability to feel for himself the discomfort that others would experience as a result of his antisocial activities that is absent in the psychopath.

This personality is found more often in males than females. He is conspicuously lacking in conscience and human sympathy. He is in many ways the opposite of the anankast. He may be meaninglessly cruel, callous and aggressive. He is often cold, rejecting social norms and showing irresponsibility in his relationships. As he ages he is less likely to be in conflict with the law and less likely to be violent, but his affectionless inability to see the consequences of his actions, and the way other people suffer because of them, remains destructive in the family and in other institutions where he may be.

He fails to learn from his experience (Craft, 1966). Feeling guilt simply means the realisation that he has been discovered in this unacceptable act, and that he will have to face the consequences. There is a failure to identify with his victim; he cannot feel the embarrassment that occurs through empathising with the suffering others experience as a result of what he does.

Whiteley (1975) has defined psychopathy as follows. The psychopath is an individual:

(1) who persistently behaves in a way which is not in accord with the accepted social norms of the culture or times in which he lives;

(2) who appears to be unaware that his behaviour is seriously at fault; and,

(3) whose abnormality cannot readily be explained as resulting from the 'madness' we commonly recognise nor from 'badness' alone.

Assessment of Personality Disorder

There are two major questions in this context. How does one determine if personality disorder is present?; and, if so, what sort of personality disorder is it? To decide whether personality disorder is present requires a judgment of what degree of severity will constitute disorder, and therefore measurement is necessary. The type of personality disorder is by no means discrete or absolute; different personality categories commonly coincide in the same person. Three further questions are then raised: If personality disorder is a life-long trait, how consistent is diagnosis at subsequent assessment? With what other states may personality disorder be confused? How does one make the distinction between neurosis and neurotic characteristics of personality?

Reliability of Diagnosis

When the presence and type of personality disorder is ascertained at different times or by a different interviewer reliability is low. This is partly because the terms used to describe types of personality have different meanings for different people, for example, 'hysterical' (Walton and Presly, 1973). Also the normal variation of personality traits is ill-defined, for example, how much 'manipulativeness' is within normal limits. Because of the impreciseness of the terms used, there will be biases, in diagnosis, for instance, in one clinic 70% of the patients were considered to have anankastic personality.

Despite these difficulties, there is a significant degree of reliability between different raters assessing personality, and also with the same rater over a 12 month interval (Tyrer *et al.*, 1979). When the same rater assessed the patient's personality after a 12-year interval, there was a significant degree of reliability for the personality trait present. This was more marked for the better defined personality traits, for example, anankastic personalities.

Similarly when inter-rater reliability was investigated for Schneider's typology for the diagnosis of personality disorder, a high level of agreement was found between three psychiatrists assessing personality under experimental conditions (Standage, 1979). The chief problem over reliability would seem to be that some patients show definite characteristics of two or more personality types. In such a case, both diagnoses should be made. The descriptions of personality types should not be considered mutually exclusive. That is, a person with anankastic personality may also show hysterical or affective traits of personality. The 'types' are descriptions of that personality in pure form; individual patients may be categorised according to the type or types which they most closely resemble.

To achieve a satisfactory level of reliability, a standardised pro-forma must be used for enquiring about personality. Tyrer *et al.* (1979) took 24 personality attributes which were relatively independent of each other and could have serious effects on social and personal adjustments when present to an abnormal degree. Each of these attributes was rated on a 9-point scale and a schedule was derived, which has proved useful in the clinical assessment of personality disorder, and gives satisfactory reliability.

A different typological scheme of assessment of abnormal personality has been introduced by Mann and Jenkins (1981) for research purposes. Reliable rating was demonstrated between different psychiatrists and this was consistent over time. It was found necessary to add 'anxious' and 'self-conscious' personalities to the list of the International Classification.

Differential Diagnosis of Personality Disorder

There is no sharp demarcation between personality disorder and normality. An operational definition has to be made to decide what personality traits will be regarded as important, how much of these characteristics will be required to constitute abnormality of personality, and what severity amounts to personality disorder.

Equally there is no clear distinction between personality disorder and neurosis, or what has been described earlier as the 'subclinical neurosis syndrome'. When previously treated neurotic patients were compared with a control group of people who had received hospital treatment for varicose veins but had no known neurotic symptomatology, at 12-year follow-up 70% of the previous neurotic group were considered to show personality disorder whereas only 25% of the non-neurotic population showed an equivalent degree of disorder of personality (Sims and Gooding, 1975). This is a high estimate of abnormality of personality but clearly there is very considerable overlap between neurosis and personality disorder.

It is important to state that not all psychopaths are criminal, nor are all criminals psychopathic. Henderson (1939) described creative, inadequate and aggressive psychopathy, citing Lawrence of Arabia as an example of a creative psychopath. The Mental Health Act (1959) states 'psychopathic disorder means a persistent disorder or disability of mind (whether or not including subnormality of intelligence) which results in abnormally aggressive or seriously irresponsible conduct on the part of a patient, and requires, or is susceptible to medical treatment'. This definition of psychopathy concentrates very much on the antisocial aspects of personality disorder, and has been modified in the Review of the Mental Health Act, 1976, 'severe personality disorder means a persistent abnormality of mind of such a kind and degree as seriously to affect the person's life or adjustment to society, and which is so marked as to render him a serious risk to himself or to others (Department of Health and Social Security, 1976).

Scott made the point that society calls a man 'psychopathic' with the implication that he is ill if it wants to treat him medically and considers that treatment may be beneficial. Society describes him as a 'recidivist' and regards him as criminal if they don't wish to treat him but simply incarcerate him. Baronness Wootton (1959) has, with admirable clarity, described psychopathic individuals as 'extremely selfish persons and no one knows what makes them so'.

This doubt about the psychopathic personality raises the question as to whether psychopathy is a useful concept at all. Walton *et al.* (1970) categorises personality disorders in different grades of severity, and this follows the hierarchical view of mental illness described by Foulds (1976). Those situations, where the disorder of personality causes other people to suffer, are regarded as the most severe type of personality disorder, and this, of course, coincides most closely with psychopathy. However, the Schneiderian concept of personality disorder reckons that personality disorder is present whenever an abnormality of personality causes the person himself or others to suffer. This could imply mild personality disorder where other people are caused to suffer to a fairly minor extent, or severe personality disorder when the person himself suffers very greatly as a result of his personality. As far as psychopathy is concerned it is best to regard it as 'asocial personality disorder' (previously described); one type of personality disorder amongst several.

There is sometimes a difficult distinction between personality disorder of affective type and affective disorders. Is the depression in this patient a temporary state of illness or a lasting trait of personality? Obviously the history and the account of premorbid personality is very important for making this distinction.

Occasionally it is very difficult to distinguish brain damage and organic states following trauma, including surgery, from personality disorders. There are specific non-psychotic mental disorders following organic brain damage. The personality may be organically damaged in such conditions and also in association with epilepsy. In these organic cases personality disorder could be considered to be secondary — pseudo — personality disorder; comparable to the secondary impairment of intelligence due to brain damage perhaps from head injury, whilst primary impairment is due to mental handicap.

Borderline states are discussed quite a lot in the American psychiatric literature. Bearing in mind our geographical analogy for neurosis in chapter 1, it is logically impossible for a *state* to be *borderline* — there could be a border *zone* state, but a line must discriminate between two distinct categories. These borderline states are supposed to lie between psychosis, especially schizophrenic psychosis, and severe neurosis but they seem to rely for their existence upon fuzziness of diagnostic criteria and upon a readiness to over-diagnose schizophrenia using a wider definition of this illness. Current European diagnosis finds this over-inclusive. Frequently, those patients diagnosed *borderline state* in North America would be regarded as severe neurosis with personality disorder in Europe.

Occasionally there may be real difficulty in distinguishing schizophrenia from personality disorder. This difficulty occurs in two situations especially. First, simple schizophrenia may be difficult to distinguish from schizoid personality where the person shows callousness, recklessness, shallow affect and lack of will or drive. One would look for a distinct break in the life history to suggest that schizophrenia is the more likely diagnosis. Second, in residual or defect state following a schizophrenic illness, there may be a deterioration of the personality.

Neurosis and Neuroticism

Neurosis is therefore the state or reaction to adverse circumstances, peculiar for each individual person but conforming to certain patterns; neuroticism is the abnormality of personality that is found to predispose to neurotic reactions. Neurosis is the description of the illness, if the term 'illness' is used, neuroticism is the background characteristic of personality of such people.

As human beings we are all different from each other and that which makes us different (apart from our physical characteristics) is called our personality. Our personality is expressed through the behaviour which we normally show; it is the sum of our aims and goals. Each person is unique, he looks, thinks and acts differently from everyone else. However, his style of reactions to situations, he holds in common with some other people. When we describe him, the adjectives we use are the description both of his personality, and of the similarities he has to some people and the differences to others. Julian Huxley has described this, 'during man's growth, mere individuality becomes personality'. William James' comment was, 'in most of us, by the age of 30, the character has set like plaster, and will never soften again'. We tend to classify people according to the characteristics (liked or disliked) that they either share or do not share with some other person we know well. Neuroticism describes a collection of attitudes of personality that predisposes to neurotic behaviour.

Bibliography

Chick, J., Waterhouse, L. and Wolff, S. (1979). Psychological construing in schizoid children grown up. *Br. J. Psychiat.*, 135, 425–430

Craft, M. (1966). *Psychopathic Disorders*, Pergamon Press, Oxford

De Alarcon, R.D. (1973). Hysteria and hysterical personality disorder. *Psychiat. Q.*, 47, 258–275

Department of Health and Social Security (1976). *A Review of the Mental Health Act*, 1959, H.M.S.O., London

Essen-Möller, E. (1956). Individual traits and morbidity in a Swedish rural population. *Acta psychiat. neurolog., Scand.* Suppl. 100

Eysenck, H.J. (1969). *The Structure and Measurement of Personality*, Routledge and Kegan Paul, London

Foulds, G.A. (1976). *The Hierarchical Nature of Personal Illness*, Academic Press, London

Henderson, D.K. (1939). *Psychopathic States*, W.W. Norton, New York

Mann, A.H. and Jenkins, R. (1981). The development and use of a standardized assessment of abnormal personality. *Psychol. Med.*, 11, 839–847

Mental Health Act (1959). 7th and 8th Edition, H.M.S.O., London

Schneider, K. (1958). *Psychopathic Personalities* (Trans. Hamilton, M.W.), Cassell, London

Sims, A.C.P. and Gooding, K. (1975). The psychiatric outcome of ' normal' people at follow-up. *Psychiat. Res.*, 12, 167-175

Sjobring, H. (1973). Personality structure and development. *Acta Psychiat. Scand.*, Supplement, 244

Standage, K.F. (1979). The use of Schneider's typology for the diagnosis of personality disorder — An examination of reliability. *Br. J. Psychiat.*, 135, 238-242

Thompson, D.J. (1980). A comprehensive study of hysterical personality disorder. Unpublished Dissertation for degrees of M.Sc., Faculty of Medicine, University of Manchester

Tyrer, P. and Alexander, J. (1979). Classification of personality disorder. *Br. J. Psychiat.*, 135, 163-7

Tyrer, P., Alexander, M.S., Cicchetti, D., Cohen, M.S. and Remington, M. (1979). Reliability of a schedule for rating personality disorders. *Br. J. Psychiat.*, 135, 168-74

Walton, H.J., Foulds, G.A. and Littmann, S.K. (1970). Abnormal personality. *Br. J. Psychiat.*, 116, 497-510

Walton, H.J. and Presly, A.S. (1973). Use of a category system in the diagnosis of abnormal personality: Dimensions of abnormal personality. *Br. J. Psychiat.*, 122, 259-276

Whiteley, J.S. (1975). The psychopath and his treatment. In: *Contemporary Psychiatry* (Ed. Silverstone, T. and Barraclough, B.), Headley Brothers, Ashford, Kent

Wootton, B.F. (1959). *Social Science and Social Pathology*, Allen & Unwin, London

World Health Organization (1977). *Manual of the International Classification of Diseases, Injuries and Causes of Death*, 9th Revision, Vol. 1, W.H.O., Geneva

8 Social Aspects of Neurosis

'Nature urges that a man should wish human society to exist and should wish to enter it.

(Cicero, De Officiis, I. iv)

'It is to the weakest and most unfortunate that society owes most diligent protection and care'.

Jean Colombier 1736–1789, quoted
R. Semelaigne, 'Les Pionniers'

In this chapter I am going to discuss a topic which is often overlooked in the description of human affairs; the interaction between the neurotic and the society in which he lives. Society impinges upon the individual and causes him to react. However, in the same sense that any of us are responsible for our behaviour, the neurotic is also. Behaviour resulting from neurotic attitudes affects a person's family, his workmates and the other people around him. This is what we will explore in this chapter.

An optician tested a patient's eyes and told her that her spectacles were satisfactory. She returned to his clinic on several subsequent weeks with trivial complaints about her vision. On about the fourth occasion he looked at her spectacles but did not test her eyesight. Later that day she telephoned him in the hospital saying, 'What do I do to make a complaint about my hospital treatment? You did not examine my eyes today'. When this most accommodating optician said, 'That is unnecessary. If you would like to come back I will certainly examine your eyes but there won't be any change in them', she replied, 'Oh no, I have a right to see someone else. I am not going to see you again. Who else can I see in the hospital?'. What was so characteristic of neurotic maladroitness in social relationships was that her request about to whom to make a complaint was addressed to the very object of her complaints.

The influential control various aspects of the lives of other people by their behaviour; many different underlying motivations have been ascribed to them: greed, desire for power, altruism, love of God, patriotism and so on. It is also recognised that some have made decisions resulting from madness, but neuroticism has rarely been invoked in history except within the rather narrow framework of Freudian theory. The effects of neurosis in public life are beyond the scope of this book, but would merit further discussion. The more influential a man is, the more his neurotic symptoms will have an effect upon others. It may be his neurotic drive which makes a man influential; the anxious thrust for domination arising from his inner insecurity.

To be deemed 'neurotic' an action must be seen as inappropriate to the person's peer group — it marks him out from his fellows. So for a primitive tribesman to wear a necklace of crocodile's teeth to ward off illness is not neurotic, if all of his tribe do the same. For an English patient to attend his general practitioner weekly for several months importuning for investigations to exclude cancer would be regarded as neurotic behaviour. It is outside social norms. The relationship between neurosis and society needs to be viewed in this way — neurosis describes individual behaviour or attitudes with social repercussions.

Neurosis occurs in all social classes but where investigated has proved to be somewhat commoner in social classes 4 and 5 than 1 and 2. However, this is difficult to estimate as criteria used for measuring frequency in different populations are not constant. As well as having more neurotic problems, those of lower social class have less easy access to treatment facilities. In many aspects of the relation between neurosis and society, neurosis both causes adverse social circumstances and results from them.

Work and Neurosis

The potentially harmful effect of unemployment upon psychological stability has been known since the work of Eisenberg and Lazarsfeld (1938). This and related studies have shown how problems associated with work and unemployment can provide the stress to precipitate a neurotic reaction (Rees, 1981). However, what is less obvious but also important is that the person who already suffers from neurosis is more at risk from various work problems.

Obtaining Work

At a time of high unemployment the neurotic person is at a disadvantage in obtaining suitable work. When applying for a post in competition with other similarly qualified applicants, personality problems may impair his performance at selection procedure, and will perhaps have damaged his reputation with his referees. He may have experienced an unhappy childhood and make choices in early adult life coloured to too great an extent by this. For example, he may join the Services, not because he sees this as the most rewarding work available to him, but solely to escape from an unhappy family. Both because he has difficulties in obtaining suitable work and because he is likely to make unsatisfactory choices, the neurotic may well establish himself at a critical period of life in his early twenties with uncongenial work making for difficulties in coping. These factors accumulate, tending towards poor performance at work, and hence an unsatisfactory work record with less job stability, more frequent change of occupation, greater likelihood of sacking or redundancy, more time off work due to sickness or unemployment, and less job satisfaction, lower pay and status resulting from work.

The Neurotic in his Role at Work

It is too easy but unjustifiable to convert terms describing the individual into metaphors used for the group, such as the 'industrial neurosis' of strikers, the 'depressive reaction' of management, the 'national malaise' which manifests itself in industrial conflict, and so on. Neurosis and depression are relevant on a national scale in industry as the problems of individuals: the neurotic is more likely to experience difficulties at work; such a person is predisposed for individual reasons to be most sensitive to the disturbance resulting from industrial conflict. Strict usage of these terms describing neurotic problems does not permit their use for a group; most workers on strike will not be suffering from neurosis, nor will most managers be clinically depressed.

It has been estimated that in the United Kingdom 37 million working days are lost per year through psychological disorder, and this exceeds the 23 million days lost through accidents at work. The former figure is an under-estimate, as it excludes physical symptoms associated with psychological disturbance. Accidents are also more likely to occur in the neurotically predisposed, and those who are neurotic and experience an accident are more likely to take time off than those without neurosis. The number of days taken off work for psychological symptoms is increasing at a more rapid rate than for other causes of sickness.

There is a tendency for those with neurosis not to be using their full intellectual abilities in their work. A university student lost a term off his course due to neurotic illness. He was allowed to complete his degree, but obtained a lower Class than expected and was not accepted for teacher training. He disliked his clerical job, found it boring, and he made no progress in achieving promotion. His three months' neurotic condition had permanently affected his career. The neurotic tends to be employed at a level too low for his abilities because, (1) he tends to obtain the wrong job for the reasons described above, and (2) when in a particular post, because of his neurotic characteristics, he fails to make the best of his job. For example, a neurotic woman in an administrative post was for ever arguing with her subordinates and so was not given the responsibility normally associated with the post.

At work one takes on a role which is institutional and not personal; for example, 'manager with responsibility for the North Eastern sales division' tells you nothing about the man himself. The role describes both the responsibilities in the job, and also the implied communication with other people. Neurotics tend to have difficulties in their work-role because they misinterpret these communications. A secretary working for a Charity was furious inside herself every time anyone came into her office to give her letters; she felt that this was treating her in an inferior way and she resented this. There is a greater tendency for the neurotic to find his work more futile than other people. He also finds 'carrying' responsibility for other people more stressful because of his problem with communication and his doubts about himself.

Job Satisfaction

Apart from financial remuneration other rewards are expected from work. Work should present some sort of mental or physical challenge capable of being overcome. For the neurotic with low self-esteem and inconsistent performance this may not represent a challenge but a threat. It is important to have a personal interest in one's work, but the anxious self-centredness of the neurotic precludes this. There should be a match between the rewards for work and the person's expectations. However, as we have already discussed there is a tendency for the neurotic to be working below his capacity and therefore his expectations also. Good working conditions are important for job satisfaction, but conditions which may be alright for others may be unsatisfactory for the neurotic because of his own problems. For example, a job involved sharing an office with one other person; after several years of congenial partnership one of the pair was replaced by a person with neurotic difficulties. The two argued so that they could not work together, and the neurotic person complained that she did not like working on her own. High self-esteem in work for the individual is important as a factor promoting job satisfaction, for example, the long serving ward cleaner who rightly knows that everyone relies upon her. This is, of course, intrinsically more difficult to achieve for a person with neurotic difficulties who comes to work with self-esteem already impaired.

The *work ethic* is sometimes commented upon in derisory terms. However, there is evidence that 'work is good for you'. Shepherd and Barraclough (1980) investigated Durkheim's theory of the protective nature of work from suicide. Seventy five people who killed themselves were matched with 150 controls; the suicides showed more unemployment before their deaths, more absence from work because of illness; they had more frequent changes of occupation, and held their jobs for shorter periods. Amongst the older subjects, suicides were less likely to have retired gradually; they were more likely to come from occupations with high risk for suicide. It is known, of course, that suicides have a high level of psychiatric morbidity before carrying out their act.

Stress at Work

Problems at work are likely to be perceived as more stressful by neurotics than by others. This is true for the physical stresses associated with noise, temperature, humidity, vibration and illumination. The neurotic is likely to be less tolerant of bad working conditions, and he may link his neurotic symptoms, for example phobia or anxiety, to problems at work. Non-physical stresses at work, for example, fear of redundancy may be more of a threat for the neurotic person who has just joined the staff following a hospital admission; especially if he finds the work uncongenial and is making poor relationships with his workmates. Fatigue is a potent stress, and so also is too little work (Cox, 1978). Various devices have been introduced in industry to try to overcome the problem of work being excessively boring, for example, giving car workers a larger number of different tasks so that they may have a greater feeling of involvement in the finished product. Work may also, of course, be too threatening; for example, an anaesthetist complained that his work was very boring for 99% of the time, but he was terrified during the other 1%. Because of his previous experience the neurotic may be unable to resolve the stresses of work in an appropriate way.

Relationships at work are likely to be difficult for the neurotic. Perhaps arising from conflict in getting on with his own parents, he may have a very uneasy relationship with his boss. He tends to misperceive the non-verbal cues in communication ('people don't look at me in the office') and he may be unduly self-referrent in the way he interprets conversations; ('they are always making snide remarks about me'). This is likely to cause difficulties with his colleagues. His self-doubts may render him incapable of dealing with subordinates at work. Sometimes the trouble maker or isolant at work has neurotic disorder, and neurotic behaviour can precipitate industrial conflict. Bad feelings in a complete working group in a firm or industry or office may result from one individual neurotic person's disturbance. The difficulties of the individual neurotic at work affect many others, and understanding this and dealing with it may be an effective way of improving conditions.

Unemployment and the Threat of Redundancy

Major life events have been quantified by Holmes and Rahe (1967) and, if those life events are scored, above a critical level a person is at greater risk of developing illness. Losing one's employment, changing to a different type of work and retirement were all found to rank high as significant life events. Loss of work is likely to increase the risk both of physical and psychiatric morbidity.

Eisenberg and Lazarsfeld (1938) recognised three phases in the response to unemployment. First was shock, denial and a sense of optimism — the person takes what he feels is a long deserved holiday. Second is distress, increasing as he finds it difficult to obtain work and experiences economic hardship. The third phase is more characteristic of neurotic depression. He develops the 'unemployed identity'; he stops looking systematically for work but becomes haphazard and dispirited and becomes quite hopeless about ever obtaining a job.

In a pilot study carried out for the Department of Health by Fagin (1981), there was shown to be a deterioration of the health of the 22 families studied. Moderate or severe depression, exacerbation of physical illness (such as psoriasis or asthma) were more likely to occur both in the ex-worker and his children. Marital relationships deteriorated and the children tended to perform worse at school.

Unemployment is, of course, associated with poverty, and not only is poverty and lower social class associated with a greater likelihood of many illnesses, but such people have less availability to treatment resources (Department of Health and Social Security, 1980). This is well illustrated with psychotherapy for the treatment of neuroses; until the relatively recent past psychotherapy was a conspicuously middle class activity.

Marital Dysfunction

Neuroticism may pervade marriage, and the similarities between neurotic and normal in the relationship tend to become more pronounced with longer duration of marriage; that is the neurotic and his spouse tend to converge (Hagnell and Kreitman, 1974). The wives of neurotic male patients spent more time in face-to-face contact with their husbands than was found in wives of a control group; they had fewer social contacts and poorer social integration, whilst wives of non-neurotics tend to increase their social contacts over the years of marriage (Kreitman *et al.*, 1970). The wives of neurotics were more neurotic themselves than the control-group wives, and this became more marked in marriages of longer duration.

Neurosis is associated with marital discord, separation and divorce. This poor marital adjustment is due to the disparity between giving and receiving affection: alternatively, this could be described as imbalance between care-giving and the need for attachment. When the frequency of mental illness in married couples was studied in Sweden, a great excess of mental illness was found in both partners in the marriage (Hagnell and Kreitman, 1974). Diagnosis was usually neurosis or personality disorder for the wives, and frequently alcoholism in the husbands.

Since about 1960 there has been a rapid increase, which is still accelerating, in the rate for divorce in Western Europe and the United States (Home Office, 1979). About 250 000 people are divorced each year in Britain and 100 000 people approach marital agencies for help. Vulnerability occurs especially within the earliest years of marriage, with nearly half of all divorces in the first 9 years. The highest rate for separation is within the first year of marriage and for divorce in the third year. Marked changes in the role of women in society and of attitudes towards marriage have contributed to the increase in breakdown. The change of attitudes towards marriage has been described by Dominian (1980) as a change from 'institution' to 'relationship'. There have been changes in the law facilitating divorce in several countries, and there has also been an increase in prosperity and longevity (with consequent increase of very long marriages) and a decrease in the number of children per family. The neurotic person is more likely to experience frequent conflict in marriage, and this is more likely to result in divorce.

Various factors associated with marital pathology occur with greater frequency, or predict a worse outcome in neurosis. The constellation of young age at marriage, premarital pregnancy, lower social class and family income and a need to share housing with other relatives predisposes to marital problems. Precipitate marriage with a brief, stormy or unhappy courtship is often followed by marital problems, as also persistent opposition to the marriage by the parents.

Symptoms of a Disordered Marriage

Diminished self-esteem erodes the ability to cope in neurosis. Because of this, expectations from relationships are blighted by past failure, and because he feels incompetent the neurotic does not build a relationship; 'to receive the care of others we need to feel lovable, and to care for others we need to feel that we have something positive to offer. As the result of an indifferent upbringing with poor or absent response from parents a person may not be able to feel lovable, wanted, or appreciated. Such a person yearns to be loved but feels unworthy of attention. Care and attention can only be earned and so he spends his life pleasing others without ever feeling good enough to be loved unconditionally. Such a person needs love badly but when he receives love he cannot register or retain it. He is generous and helpful in order to please others but in return feels used rather than appreciated. He is intensely angry with those close to him on whom he relies for his survival. Alternatively he feels so needy that his very needs make him feel bad. When anyone tries to reach him he withdraws because he feels that his excessive need will be experienced as greed or selfishness and his anger over his deprivation punished with further rejection' (Dominian, 1980).

Lack of self-esteem is a major bar to an equal, giving relationship in marriage. Also a chronic need to be appreciated by other people may be manifested as excessive dependence which strains the marital bond. Alternatively, attempting to deal with conflict by extreme self-sufficiency which prevents any sort of close relationship developing may damage the relationship. There may be problems in the ability to trust; this may show itself in anxious attachment. This was exemplified by a husband who was always checking up on his wife, not as a manifestation of morbid jealousy but simply because he was afraid all the time that he might lose her. Lack of trust may also show itself in a studied callousness, demonstrating no apparent need for the other partner. Learning how to form emotional bonds occurs early in childhood and longstanding disturbance of the ability to make relationships may be due to a defect at this stage. Sometimes when the spouse is lost at separation or divorce, anxious searching and panic, as is more usual in bereavement, may be shown.

Marriage problems are amongst the commonest symptoms that neurotic patients describe. Sometimes classically neurotic symptoms, for example, agoraphobia are presented first but, as these remit and the patient gets to know her doctor better, marital problems which originally were denied take the fore. Such a wife may describe her husband as 'golden' because of his resigned toleration of her neuroticism, but despite a relationship in which arguing does not take place there are frustrations and resentments in the marriage, and the wife feels unable to express her feelings, or be herself. There is a tendency for neurotic people to marry each other, and also for inappropriate behaviour arising from one partner's neuroticism to be the stress provoking neurotic symptoms in the other partner. Sometimes the choice of partner is an inappropriate way of trying to make up for long lasting deficiencies in the individual. Such misguided union may well end with breakdown.

Marital problems are rarely presented to the doctor straight-forwardly. Other symptoms are described first and only in discussion do the difficulties within the marriage loom large. Any of the whole gamut of neurotic, psychosomatic, or drug and alcohol-dependent symptoms may be associated with marital dysfunction, because there is such a close link between the presence of neurosis and marital difficulty. Insomnia is particularly frequent, as are also depression and anxiety. Somatic complaints are common, for example, abdominal pains, headache, frequency of micturition, dyspareuria and backache. While the wife is likely to present with psychosomatic symptoms, the husband often denies his marriage problems by escaping into the solace of alcohol excess. More than half of alcoholic men by the time they receive treatment are already separated or divorced. Problems in the marriage are both a result of the excess drinking and also a cause of it.

Attempted suicide is extremely common following marital difficulties. In a study of self-poisoning, 68% of married man and 60% of married women described marital disharmony as the major precipitating factor (Kessel, 1965). Thirty per cent of the marriages of the men and 26% of the women had broken down and in 17% the break up had been within a month of the suicidal attempt. In a study of parasuicide from Oxford (Bancroft et al., 1977) a decade later an even higher proportion of married men and women complained of marital problems. Half of the married men described an extramarital affair in the previous 12 months; very frequently a quarrel had preceded the suicidal attempt by a few days, and was considered to have provoked the act. Separation was also found to be an important precipitant.

Completed suicide is also related to marital difficulties; an established marriage relationship offers some protection against suicide. The suicide rate is lowest for the married proportion of the population; it is higher for those who are single or widowed; it becomes considerably higher for those who are divorced; and highest of all for those married but living apart — that is, those whose marital difficulties have not been resolved one way or the other are most likely to kill themselves. For those who are married, childlessness appears to increase the risk of suicide, as does instability of the marriage. When one partner is ill the risk of suicide to the other partner is only increased when the ill partner is in hospital.

Problems of personality are a potent source of difficulty in marriage, either in provoking disharmony or becoming manifest because of marriage problems. The person with paranoid, self-referrent personality tends to bear a grudge and feels that the other partner is deliberately flouting his wishes. Males of this type may be aggressive and sometimes violent; females are more likely to nag, and be the victims of violence.

The dysthymic or depressive personality may be a miserable, ill-tempered person to live with, and the partner may eventually be unable to tolerate any more of his partner's persistent gloom. Similarly the partner may be unable to tolerate the excessive and unpredictable swings of mood of the cyclothymic personality.

The schizoid personality conveys his emotional remoteness from human beings; to his partner he is callous, affectionless and indifferent, with no need for close relationship. Conversely, the dependent, passive personality, whether he be asthenic and inadequate relying wholly upon his wife, or whether she be histrionic, emotionally shallow and labile, may destroy the marriage by making excessive demands on the other partner who finds himself unable to shoulder all the responsibilities of the family. The insensitiveness and lack of understanding for the effects of his behaviour makes the person with asocial personality disorder a poor marriage partner.

The obsessional, controlling personality is very difficult to live with on an equal basis, and although such a personality is unlikely to break the marriage contract from his side, he may provoke the other partner by his extreme rigidity being more than she can abide.

A particular type of neurotic disorder, engagement neurosis (engyesis), occurs most often in those of obsessional personality. The person feels oppressed by the responsibility invested in his or her marriage and is filled with doubts as to whether he has made the right decision. Quite frequently he vacillates throughout the engagement with severe episodes of anxiety and misery. Usually these cases resolve on either marriage or breakage of the engagement. In some cases the symptoms of obsessional and sensitive personality continue in a different form after marriage.

Environmental Factors

The neurotic is prone to the same external stresses as other people, but predisposed to react adversely to them. Finance is a common source of argument in marriage; the wife may feel that her husband is not providing adequately for the family, or the husband may consider his wife to be a spendthrift. With blurring of the traditional roles in marriage, financial conflicts still exist, but become altered in their content, for example, a husband whose wife was earning more than he became envious of his wife, and made things difficult for her at work so that she lost her job.

Problems may involve work and marriage and a person who is already experiencing neurotic illness will find these problems a more severe source of conflict. The husband (more often) may find his time is absorbed by work, and his wife feels neglected, or even in competition with his work for time and attention. Similarly the wife giving up a career to look after young children may feel cheated and look enviously at her husband whom she feels has a congenial life compared with hers. Occasionally with her husband's promotion, the wife feels ill at ease in the new social role imposed upon her.

Relationships with the family of the other partner, particularly, of course, mother-in-law, can cause conflict. A frequent area of dispute is the division of labour in the home; with changing roles, it is not clear within the household which tasks should be done by whom, and frequently one or other partner feels imposed upon. There are many problems associated with sexual dysfunction, or the use of sex as a bargaining point within marriage, and this latter can be seen as neurotic in that it is ultimately inappropriate in achieving goals. Lack of emotional understanding is frequently levelled at husbands as a criticism, and not infrequently the husband feels that his wife does not understand his needs.

Sometimes one spouse has a neurotic need to look after a sick person, and marries the other because of his handicap. His recovery may frustrate her need for this dependence. Occasionally this is seen with the wife of an alcoholic husband who requires her husband to be delinquent and economically dependent, although, of course, more often the situation is that she would be only too delighted for her husband to stop drinking and take his share of responsibility in the family.

Conflict over diverse educational and intellectual interests occurs, especially when there are great disparities in these areas. It is very difficult for a couple to know how the other partner will react to being a parent, and frequently disagreement arises because one partner has a completely different approach to child-rearing from his spouse. This often reflects the differences in their own upbringing. Religious and spiritual difficulties quite frequently occur. These may be based upon belonging to different religions, but also upon the different ways they experience or practise their faith.

Problems in the marriage of parents is a precipitant for various difficulties in the children. Young children may show emotional and physical symptoms with patterns of disturbed behaviour. Conduct disorders are commonly associated with severe parental disharmony, and similarly difficulties in the marriage and separation are frequent antecedents for delinquency in children.

Problems of the Unmarried

Neurotic symptoms may be provoked by dissatisfaction with the unmarried state. This is most common in unmarried women, who traditionally designated a passive role in courtship, in their early thirties feel anxious that they are 'on the shelf'. Single men are more likely to show symptoms a decade later associated with doubts about sexual orientation, hypochondriacal neurosis and fears of loneliness. Neurotic symptoms are frequent with depression, anxiety, irritability and problems experienced in what were previously quite satisfactory relationships.

As she sees her previous female friends and sisters marrying and starting families, the single woman may become upset and envious. She is torn between wanting to be with young children and at the same time wanting to avoid them because of her complicated mixture of feelings; missing out, rejection, loss, a spectator of life. In order to resolve this conflict she may marry precipitately an unsuitable partner. Finding satisfaction and fulfilment in work and other activities, especially if these are emotionally and intellectually demanding and involve helping other people, has often been found to be the most successful way to sublimate these feelings for those who do not marrry.

The most important need of those in such a predicament is to feel that they belong. The greatest requirement is to be a valued, preferably essential, member of a community; ideally this will be two interlocking communities, both the family, where they will have a respected and valued place, and a larger society which might be the village, the church, a local voluntary group, social club or their function at work. Because they do not necessarily have such an established place in a social group through marriage, they may have to work at it quite hard, and the neurotic because of difficulties in relating may fail to achieve this successful integration.

Sexual Pathology

Sexual difficulties occur, of course, in people without neurotic problems, but neurosis may provoke symptoms of sexual disorder, and it may also render a person more likely to complain of existing problems. Sexual pathology will be discussed under two categories; sexual dysfunction and sexual deviation.

There are varying degrees of sexual difficulty in the female, from slight reticence in intercourse with low libido to complete orgasmic failure and vaginismus. Impotence in a male implies either erectile impotence or premature ejaculation. Commonly fear of failure associated with a very short-lived erection prevents the possibility of satisfactory intercourse. There are many causes of diminished libido in the male, such as psychiatric disorder, marital dysfunction, any type of life stress, and alcohol excess — any of these causes may be associated with neurosis. Sexual dysfunction is an important cause of marital discord.

The boundaries between normal sexual behaviour and what is regarded as abnormal or deviant are not precise, and are affected by external circumstances; for example, homosexual behaviour became common amongst troops confined to an island for a year without access to women. In this context Scott (1964) has defined the characteristics of deviant behaviour: 'the elements of a comprehensive definition of sexual perversion should include sexual activity or fantasy directed towards orgasm other than genital intercourse with a willing partner of the opposite sex and of similar maturity, persistently recurrent, not merely a substitute for preferred behaviour made difficult by the immediate environment and contrary to the generally accepted norm of sexual behaviour in the community'. The more frequent categories of sexual deviation include; (1) those where the sexual object is abnormal and (2) those where the type of sexual behaviour is abnormal (Wakeling, 1979). Of the first category are male and female homosexuality, sexuality with immature partners of either sex (paedophilia), dead people (necrophilia), animals (bestiality), or inanimate objects (fetishism), which is the experience of erotic sexual arousal associated with objects which are not normally of sexual significance, and incest (sexual behaviour with a proscribed relative). Such conditions as sadism, masochism, sexual violence and rape, exhibitionism and voyeurism are of the second category; that is, the sexual behaviour is abnormal.

Transsexualism is primarily a disorder of self-image rather than a sexual disorder. The male transsexual may regard himself as 'a female person locked inside a male body'. If he lives as a female, in feminine work, wearing female clothes, cohabiting with a male, his sexual behaviour is actually homosexual, but he does not see it this way himself because of his firmly fixed female gender identity. He strives life long to be regarded and accepted as a woman.

A clear distinction should be made between the specific abnormality of self-image in transsexualism and the purely descriptive term of transvestism; that is, the wearing of clothes appropriate to the other sex (Brierley, 1979). Transvestism occurs in theatrical female impersonators, in those who cross-dress for homosexual erotic gratification, in fetishism associated with masturbation or heterosexual behaviour, as a part of exhibitionism, and for deception in crime or espionage. Transvestism occurs also as an intermediate stage between full transsexualism and normality; such a person may feel more comfortable and at ease wearing female underclothes although these are concealed by normal male attire.

Neurosis is more frequent amongst those showing sexual deviation; this is partly because neurotics are more likely to find inappropriate sexual outlet in deviation, and partly because the stigma of deviation provokes quite frequently neurotic reaction. Not all those showing deviation manifest abnormality of personality.

The Neurotic Family and the Community

Development of the Family

What are the effects of neurotic parents upon their children? The influences and pressures parents exert will reflect their own neuroticism. Children form their standards, the viewpoint from which they assess the world outside the family, their value judgments of people, institutions and circumstances very largely upon the attitudes of their parents. They may take a similar attitude, or they may rebel against their parents' views and take a diametrically opposed position; parental influence is equally evident in both of these reactions. If the parents' behaviour is dominated by neurotic fears and limitations, this is likely to be transferred to the children.

Neurotic problems arising within families may also be seen in terms of different members' needs for attachment. Parents give care to their children; the children need to form attachment bonds and learn how to make and maintain affectionate relationships. Parents also have needs for attachment; sometimes they are inadequately met through deficiencies in care-giving by the other partner or excessive demands of the subject, and then the child becomes involved in the search for attachment of his parent. This may take different forms but all tending towards the child being brought up in a neurotic environment. A young wife and mother doted on her 6-year-old son whom she dressed in smart and rather adult clothes. Her husband was in the Merchant Navy. It was noted that when her husband was at sea, her son was kept off school for most of the time with a succession of minor illnesses. It became clear that she was using her little boy for support, he was almost literally 'in his father's shoes'.

Modelling is an important part of the development of the child.

The small boy's earliest model for what he construes to be adult male behaviour is, in the case of a complete family, his father, and so he practises being an adult by mimicking (and also emulating) his father. This will, of course, include both the socially appropriate and the neurotic behaviour of his father.

The communication system within the family is altered by the neuroticism of a prominent member. For example, a neurotic sister interprets as disparaging an innuendo from her brother when no criticism was intended. Remarks made are wrenched out of context and applied with derogatory meaning, becoming the source of acrimony and paraded as 'evidence' for years.

More specific neurotic behaviour may be transferred to the rest of the family; for example, a mother with thunder phobia is likely to communicate this to her child; in fact it is unusual to find such a fear in a child unless the mother is also afraid. Other anxieties and fears may be characteristic of a particular family, arising from one or other parent, for instance, fears concerning contamination and cleanliness, fears of particular groups of people.

We have in an earlier chapter discussed the genetic element in neurosis. It is undervalued at the present time, when genetics referred to human beings has taken on political and pejorative overtones. Genetic influences are obscured by features of early learning within the family. It is known that neurotic traits tend to concentrate within certain families, for example, obsessional or anxious predisposition. This becomes part of the consistent repertoire within the family, arising when one or other parent shows this pattern of behaviour.

Conflict in the Family

Conflict commonly occurs in the relationships of neurotics and therefore within their families. These conflicts may be openly expressed, or they may be covert, implied and only half understood by those involved. What makes them distinctively neurotic is their complete failure to resolve practical differences of opinion. In a non-neurotic argument, discussion with the opposing points of view propounded logically proceeds to resolution which may be a compromise, or a straight win for one party, or even a mutually agreed breakdown in relationship. The neurotic conflict never reaches this healthy state of definition but goes on causing misunderstanding and hurt feelings interminably. It may occur in marriage about child rearing between two parents. They may treat their children differently, not because of the variation amongst the children, but as part of working through their own neurotic attitudes. This may then produce further conflict between the siblings themselves.

Because of the neurotic's insecurity about himself, and his anxiety for survival as an independent person, his interests are centred upon himself to an excessive extent. This creates within the family an atmosphere of selfishness and hostility rather than mutual cooperation and trust. The communications of the neurotic tend to be ambiguous and he interprets other people's remarks in an oblique and deprecating way. This establishes further misunderstanding and argument.

The neurotic family atmosphere, described above, associated with the experience of an unhappy childhood tends to be communicated to the next generation, and results in the continuation of neurotic behaviour. Because of his unhappy experience in his original family, the neurotic may leave the family as soon as possible by early marriage in order to escape rather than for any positive aspects of the relationship with his wife. This then sets the scene for the establishing of another neurotic family. Neurotic choices tend to set up the situation for making further neurotic choices.

Non-accidental injury inflicted on children by their parents is often associated with parental neurosis (Smith *et al.*, 1973). For some children who are physically injured and in whom the nature of the injury is not consistent with the account of how it occurred, there is suspicion, or even more definite evidence, that the injury was inflicted by the person looking after the child. This is most common when the child is aged under 6 months. The mother more frequently causes injury, but father or other male person in the household may be implicated. Seventy six per cent of the mothers of children with non-accidental injury were found at interview following the event to have abnormal personality, and nearly half had borderline intelligence or less. Fathers frequently showed personality disorder of asocial type. The parents often described an unhappy childhood with abuse by their own parents, and feelings of rejection by and anger towards their own family. Both partners tended to share this background, with dissatisfaction within their present relationship, feelings of failure and isolation, and frequent recourse to violence. The couple tended to change partners and move house quite often, and frequently had no relatives or friends upon whom they could depend. The mother was usually young, with an unplanned pregnancy, resulting in this child; the parents were frequently unmarried at the time of the child's birth. Following delivery of the child the mother was often unresponsive, showing emotional and social problems during the puerperium. The characteristic picture is, therefore, one of neurosis and social deprivation combined with personality disorder.

Neurosis and the Local Social Structure

As well as those within the family, other relationships suffer. The social network of people with neurosis, as described by Henderson and Duncan-Jones (1978) is impaired. They looked at the 'primary group' of neurotic patients and a control group. The primary group includes 'those with whom one has both interaction and commitment'; that is, all kin, nominated friends, work associates and neighbours. They found that neurotic patients were significantly deficient in the numerical size, and the affective quality of interaction with members of their primary group, and that this deficiency was greatest in relation to the principal attachment figure, such as the spouse or parent. They described a poorer quality of relationship than normal people with more argument and discord, and less feelings of satisfaction from their contact with others. They have fewer relations, not as many friends and the time they spend with other people is less than for non-neurotic people. There is in fact a poverty of human relationships.

The very meaning of *friendship* seeems to be different for the neurotic. This was exemplified in a study in which a number of neurotics were asked the question, 'Do you have any/many friends?'. This quite reasonable question was frequently misinterpreted by neurotic patients who gave answers such as 'No, I am not a busybody, I mind my own business'. Another thought the question was enquiring obliquely about homosexuality. Quite often neurotics have good friends, but their relationship is one of dependence; sustaining the relationship is hard work for the other person who has to do all the giving in the friendship rather than mutual consideration. Some neurotic people escape from their dislike of themselves and their difficulties in sustaining close exclusive relationships by making innumerable very superficial friendships.

It is common for neurotics to take their troubles to churches and their ministers, depending upon their religious affiliation. Traditionally, the Church has sustained those in need. In our society absolute economic poverty is uncommon, but the 'poor in spirit' remain. If there were not a number of people with problems in the congregation, the Church would not be fulfilling its function. It tends to attract those with emotional and psychological problems, and it is right that this should be so. It is not that the Church produces these problems in normal people, but that people with existing difficulties are attracted to a place where they hope they can find help. The neurotic often makes great demands upon the Minister's time requiring emotional support and understanding. It is characteristic for the neurotic to have frequent changes of enthusiasm, to become disillusioned with one church or sect and move to another with a different flavour. Such people can also be creative but they demand a great deal of support from the Church.

The more manipulative and socially involved neurotic plays an active part in clubs, societies and political organisations. They seek prominence and the dominance of others, perhaps to work out their sense of failure experienced at home or work. Because of their difficulties in relationships they are likely to be in conflict with other people, especially others who also have neurotic problems.

Pathological Dependence

Various types of self-destructive behaviour are based upon excessive dependence. Dependent behaviour is initiated voluntarily, but it becomes habit forming so that the person becomes unable to restrain himself even though it is damaging. It may destroy physical health, or social relationships, or both. We will discuss briefly alcoholism, drug dependence, smoking, gambling, and dependence on other people. Neurosis is an important part of this pattern. For example, Lindegard (1980) in a series of papers has pointed out the association between depression and anxiety in middle-aged people in Gothenberg, and excessive alcohol intake and decline in social class.

Alcohol and Drugs

Alcoholism is the intermittent or continuous ingestion of alcohol leading to physical, social or psychological dependence and harm. Paton and Saunders (1981) considered the following five criteria to indicate alcohol dependence; consumption of more than 80 g alcohol daily, tolerance with blood alcohol levels of more than 150 mg/100 ml, withdrawal symptoms, continual drinking in spite of psychological, social and physical problems, and abnormal blood tests. Although alcoholism is sometimes regarded as a disease, the patient's motivation is always of importance, his feelings of responsibility for himself, and his strength of character; it is vital that these aspects be considered when treatment is instigated (Davies, 1979). The alcoholic's pattern of drinking has altered so that he is drinking more heavily than other people in his peer group; the 'round' at the bar does not come fast enough for him, or perhaps he starts drinking spirits in large amounts. His daily consumption of alcohol becomes habitually heavy with little variation from day to day. When problems arise in the family, or at work, or he is charged with an offence because of his heavy drinking, he is unable to decrease it.

At times of personal stress he has recourse to relief drinking; that is he uses alcohol as an anxiolytic, elevator of mood or sedative (Glatt, 1974). He then increases his regular intake, and experiences a need for alcohol. Drink becomes very important to him; he is thinking much of the time how he can obtain his next drink. His control over drinking becomes impaired, for example, he may leave an important meeting prematurely in order to get to the bar at opening time. Occasionally he feels guilty about drinking, but often makes excuses to himself and to others. His efforts to control his drinking repeatedly fail; there is further impairment of work and loss of other interests; increasingly his life is centred upon alcohol. Although personality disorder is frequently found in alcoholism, it should not be thought that this is invariable.

Physical and psychological symptoms of dependence are present. Withdrawal symptoms occur as the level of alcohol in his blood drops. Tremor of the hands with nausea, amnesia and a feeling of apprehensiveness occurs about 8-12 hours after stopping drinking; alcohol-withdrawal fits may occur after 24-48 hours; and delirium tremens with an impaired state of consciousness, auditory and visual hallucinations and a mood of utter terror may happen between about 48 hours and 5 days after ceasing drinking. Tolerance occurs, so that a larger amount of alcohol is required to produce the same psychological state. At the same time as these biological symptoms are developing, there may be increasing social difficulties. He has more problems with money, and with his family. Loss of job and permanent breakdown of marriage frequently results from alcoholism.

Drug dependence pharmacologically and symptomatically has many similarities to alcoholism. However those involved are different in terms of age and social type. Alcoholics are more often male than female; by the time of recognition usually middle-aged; their attitude to society is generally conformist. Commonly the narcotics addict or multiple drug abuser is younger, of either sex, and identifies with a peer group opposed to society. Narcotic addicts who had stopped using drugs, when compared with those still addicted at 7-year follow-up were more likely to have a job and legitimate source of income, to be in good health and to have a stable address, and less likely to have problems with the law (Oppenheimer et al., 1979). There is a large number of people who show neurotic behaviour and who have become dependent upon prescribed drugs, especially hypnotics and minor tranquillisers. Prominent amongst these used to be the barbiturate group of drugs until their much more restricted prescription; now emotional dependence is frequently seen with the benzodiazepine drugs.

At follow-up of a cohort of previously treated neurotic patients,

10% were found to be significantly dependent upon alcohol or drugs (Sims, 1975). Those with a more severe degree of neurosis at the time of initial treatment were more likely to show dependence at the time of follow-up. Alcohol or drug dependence is one of the possible unfavourable outcomes likely to follow severe neurosis. Another type of abuse particularly prominent amongst neurotics is self-poisoning with an excess of drugs prescribed either for the patient or a relative. This behaviour is often associated with other evidence of neurotic disorder or personality problem. This is discussed in more detail later.

Other Forms of Dependence

In 1977 approximately 48% of working people in England and Wales of both sexes were regular smokers. There is a tendency for a greater proportion of neurotics to be smokers than non-neurotics; those neurotics who smoke, smoke more cigarettes than other people; they start smoking at a younger age; and a higher proportion inhale deeply (Salmons and Sims, 1981). Although social factors are often important in the initiation of smoking, its continuation at a high level may result from neurotic patterns of behaviour. The experience of smoking clinics is that this is a very difficult condition to treat.

Pathological gambling describes the situation where the gambler himself or his relatives feel gambling is excessive (Moran, 1975). He usually has an urge which is experienced as tension and only relieved by gambling. He thinks about gambling a lot of the time. Once he has started he may not be able to stop himself until all his money has gone. He may damage himself economically or socially by losing his job or harming his family. He may become depressed. Despite this the gambler has a quite unjustified belief that next time he will win (as in Dostoievsky's short story — *The Gambler*). Gambling may occur on the basis of personality disorder or neurosis; equally the damage resulting may precipitate a neurotic depressive reaction. Other neurotic behaviour such as drug overdose is common amongst pathological gamblers.

Excessive personal dependence may be formed upon those close to a neurotic person, for example upon spouse, other relative, employer, teacher, or minister. Neurotics also tend to be excessively dependent and make heavy demands upon their family doctor. This was demonstrated in examining the general practitioner case notes of neurotic patients referred to hospital when compared with a control group from the same practice. The neurotic patients' notes were of very much higher mean weight!

One group of neurotic patients who have extreme difficulty in relationships show their dependence upon institutions rather than individuals. This is characteristic of the Munchausen Syndrome (Asher, 1951) with repeated admissions to hospital and importunate requests for treatment. The illness-behaviour shown both by those with hysteria and those with hypochondriasis is a neurotic manifestation of excessive dependence.

Welfare departments and social security organisations, simply through being bureaucratic bodies, are clumsy at helping individuals to cope better, especially when that individual is as sensitive as the neurotic. Support can very easily be counter-productive, reinforcing the patient's attitude of impotent helplessness rather than encouraging him towards independence. Handouts of money which the person knows he has not earned is against sound psychological principle in the management of neurosis; it establishes dependence upon the authorities and provides no motivation to improve his own situation. Financial support is undoubtedly necessary and therefore more therapeutic methods of distribution are required.

Social Neuroses

The conditions under which people live has clearly a lot to do both with their development of neurosis and the form that neurotic illness takes. Particular situations of society as they affect individual people are likely to provoke neurotic reactions; for example, economic depression and war. There is no evidence that these situations produce a higher rate of neurosis, but the content of the neurotic conflict reflects these background conditions. During a time of high unemployment, a patient became so anxious that she might be made redundant that she was unable to go to work; without social work intervention her apprehensive inertia and fear would undoubtedly have been self-fulfilling. It has been claimed that during war-time the rate for neurosis decreased. This may be an artefact of referral and facilities for treatment; during war doctors are less likely to give time for treating the neurotic, and patients are less likely to consult. During economic depression many people are anxious and fear for their jobs and their financial position. Understandably those who are neurotically predisposed will suffer these symptoms to a greater extent, so that it may become disabling.

Housing Conditions

Some aspects of neurosis are associated with living conditions. Subclinical neurosis syndrome was found in about one third of the population of a new town, in an inner city borough, and in an overspill suburb. However, different social classes, different types of environment and different ages do produce a differing range of symptoms. The housebound housewife typically is a young married woman with young children living in modern council property or new owner-occupied housing development. The female alcoholic is more often older, middle class and neglected by or separated from her husband who is, perhaps, totally absorbed by his business involvements.

There has been considerable interest in the effects of high rise dwellings on mental health. It has been claimed that the number of floors up in such a building correlates positively with the degree of psychological and social symptoms (Fanning, 1967). More recently this has been challenged (Moore, 1974), and it would seem that, as in other areas of neurosis, individual factors are all important. Young families are considerably disadvantaged by living in high rise dwellings; the young mother cannot easily get her children outside to play; she is very liable to become housebound and any disturbance in the amenities of the tower block, like a broken lift, increases her difficulties. The important factor, therefore, for the development of neurosis is how the person and family themselves regard living in a flat at a great height. The design of such living should include more than engineering and practical planning. It should be directed to the establishing of a harmonious social group (Sims, 1982). This will involve opportunity for meeting neighbours socially on neutral ground and the instilling of pride of ownership for some of the shared facilities like staircases and entrance foyers.

In this short section one can only summarise that housing conditions are relevant to the development of neurosis. Association between type of housing and presentation of symptoms needs to be explored further.

Aftermath Neurosis

To be a victim in catastrophe is extremely stressful and has a massive short-term and long-term effect upon mental equilibrium. There are two mechanisms that could explain the emotional reactions that follow involvement in major disaster. First, there is the experience of loss which is known to provoke neurosis; loss of health, loss of relatives, loss of property, loss of status. Second there is the experience of having played a passive role in the collective drama of the catastrophe. This feeling of involvement in the disaster is greater the

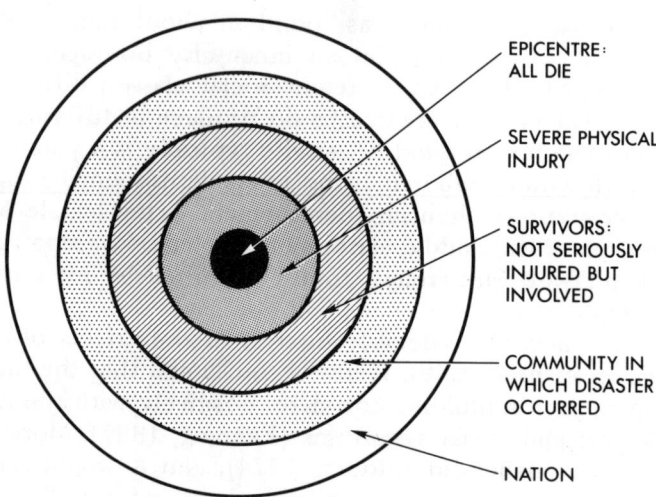

EPICENTRE:
ALL DIE

SEVERE PHYSICAL
INJURY

SURVIVORS:
NOT SERIOUSLY
INJURED BUT
INVOLVED

COMMUNITY IN
WHICH DISASTER
OCCURRED

NATION

Figure 8.1   Aftermath of disaster

closer the person was to its source (figure 8.1). At the epicentre of
a major disaster all will die. In the area adjacent to this most people
will be severely injured. Somewhat further away people will be
involved in the disaster in that they were there, but may not themselves be seriously physically injured. A distinct boundary between
those involved and the community in which the disaster occurs
increases the feeling of involvement and separation from others of
the victims. With aerial bombardment of a town the whole community
will feel involved and there is no barrier; with an explosion in a
building, those inside are quite precisely discriminated from those
outside the building who feel disturbed by the event but are not
directly involved. In the latter case those inside the building, even if
they are not injured, will feel themselves to be victims and somehow
separated from the community outside.

This was exemplified by the bomb blasts occurring in two Birmingham public houses in 1974 (Sims *et al.*, 1979). Twenty one people
were killed and 43 people were severely injured. 116 more people
were inside the two public houses at the time of the explosion;
they were taken to Casualty Departments at hospitals in the city but
were released later that evening with either no injury at all or only
slight physical disability. Understandably, they felt themselves to be
both victims and survivors, and were clearly very much involved in the
disaster, although in most instances they experienced no personal
loss. Long term neurotic disability with phobic anxiety symptoms,
irritability and depression protracted over many months, and some-

times for years, was found at follow-up. In several instances previous moderate to heavy drinking had increased to the level of definite alcohol dependence. Many of these victims claimed that their subsequent separation and divorce could be ascribed, at least in part, to the effects of the disaster. They also described problems with employment with considerable time off work due to sickness following the bombing, frequent changes of occupation in order to leave the city centre and work nearer their home, and problems in carrying out their work adequately.

These uninjured victims of disaster were compared with a matched group of people who had attended casualty departments and been allowed home the same evening but were not involved in a major catastrophe. In the six months before their accident the casualty attenders had had nearly twice as many days off work as the bomb victim group, probably because they included amongst their number regular casualty attenders with high morbidity. In the six months following the accident, the control group showed a minimal increase in days off work due to sickness, but the bomb victims suffered an eight and a half fold increase. Initial incapacity, that is days off work immediately following the accident, was enormously increased in the bomb blast group. It would seem therefore that much greater disability follows involvement in major disaster with minimal injury than from ordinary accidents occurring in individuals.

There are distinct stages in the reaction to disaster (Tyhurst, 1951) (figure 8.2). In the recoil stage the victims are often numbed and apathetic; they may show acute panic reactions or inappropriate apathetic and automatic behaviour. In their social relations soon

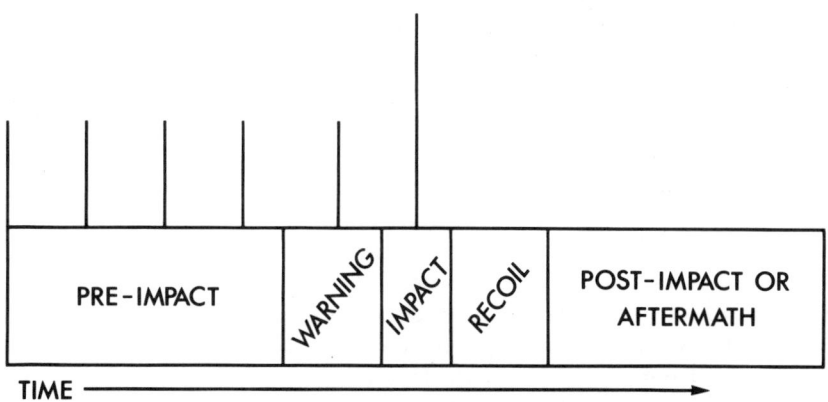

Figure 8.2   Stages of psychological reaction to disaster

after the disaster, people become helpful and cooperative towards each other, and a number of old quarrels are resolved (the post-disaster Utopia). Then quite rapidly this state of benevolence vanishes and the hostile divisions in the community once more recur. The phase of post-impact or aftermath continues for a long time, perhaps for many years (Kinston and Rosser, 1974). Aftermath neurosis occurs in that, those exposed to great stress and predisposed by personality, domestic or occupational problems, are likely to show a prolonged neurotic reaction following involvement in major disaster.

Communicated Neurosis

Neurosis may be contagious in a psychological sense; that is close contact with an individual who has symptoms may result in the transmission of symptoms to somebody previously unaffected. This tends to occur either through the powerful influence of long-term cohabitation with one other person or alternatively through the volatile collective emotions of a group — mass hysteria. A woman shared her husband's belief that he was being followed by people at work who were inserting bugging devices in their living room wall to alter his thinking. When apart from her husband for a time during his hospital admission for a psychotic illness, she realised that his story was symptomatic of his illness. Specific forms of behaviour may also be communicated, for example, in the occasional outbreaks of epidemic self-incendiarism which occur; the news media probably serve as vectors.

Epidemic, communicated or mass neurosis or insanity is transmitted through a large number of people, usually in a closed community. When physical symptoms such as hyperventilation or fainting are prominent it justifies the term *mass hysteria*. Spread occurs first via the emotionally unstable and those already experiencing considerable conflict; thus the transmission is psychological and neurotic rather than obeying laws such as occur with epidemic infection.

Such epidemics have been described throughout history, for example, the millenial movements of the middle ages described by Cohn (1957). Popular semi-educated preachers caught the imagination of the poor and dispossessed in the slums of medieval central European cities and led their followers out onto the tops of hills where they confidently expected the Second Coming to begin. These movements were associated with socially disruptive behaviour and also physical symptoms in those affected.

An epidemic spreading through a school in Blackburn was described by Moss and McEvedy (1966). Symptoms of overbreathing, dizziness, fainting, headache, shivering, pins and needles, nausea, pain in the back or abdomen, hot feelings and general weakness occurred. Such epidemics almost always occur in young females; they often start with a girl of high status in her peer group who is unhappy; they tend to occur in largest numbers in the younger children in a secondary school, that is those about puberty; and to affect those who on subsequent testing appeared to be most unstable. Isolation of those affected appears to be the best method of stopping the epidemic; for example, in an epidemic amongst nurses, sending those with symptoms home rather than keeping them together in a sick bay ended the outbreak.

Many different transcultural forms of hysteria have been described in which social pressures are clear precipitants, for example, latah (Kiev, 1972). This has a number of different names and slightly different forms in various communities in South East Asia, but characteristic is hypersuggestibility, automatic obedience, speaking obscenities, and various echo phenomena. It occurs in lower social class women exposed to sudden overwhelming stress and can be considered an acute catastrophic reaction. War, natural disasters or drastic social change are then the trigger for such a reaction; it is equivalent to aftermath neurosis described above.

A more insidious and less acute epidemic is the recent increase in the frequency of anorexia nervosa in many western affluent societies. This appears to be associated, in part, with social pressures to slim. Where food is abundant, fatness is no longer associated with being rich and successful. The pursuit of thinness has become a goal for many adolescent girls and some of these fear that they will lose their control over eating and body weight, and so they become overtly anorexic.

Institutional Neurosis

This term was introduced by Barton in 1956, and it came to be used not only to describe behaviour resulting from institutionalisation, but also the long-term defect state of mental illness. The total institution can have a destructive effect upon the spontaneity of behaviour and relationships (Goffman, 1961). It is important to realise that people with psychotic illness may have secondary neurotic disability arising either from their own perception of illness, or as a result of the conditions of treatment. Barton found similarity between the mental state of long stay patients in mental hospitals and prisoners in a concentration camp.

Characteristic of institutional neurosis are the following features: extreme apathy, lack of initiative to carry out any activities at all, loss of interest both in the environment and also in planning for the future. A prominent feature is submissiveness towards those in authority who, in the hospital setting, include all grades of staff from the most senior to the most junior nurses. Posture is described as characteristic for these subjects; the hands are held in a position of uselessness across the body, the shoulders are droppped and the head is stooped forwards and downwards with the eyes looking downwards and averted from other people. There is restriction of the arm movements associated with walking, shuffling gait (both of which can also occur as side-effects of commonly used antipsychotic drugs), and loss of expression of emotion. When criticised, the person offers no defence and expresses no resentment. He accepts his situation with resignation and does nothing to alter its course. Despite occasional outbursts of frustration, he appears to have lost all individuality. This description is not unique to hospital patients or sufferers from psychosis. It occurs in other situations, such as prison, and, when the patient is dominated by authoritarian relatives, even at home. Amongst neurotics it is those with asthenic personality who are most likely to show this reaction, but it is of course sensitive to social circumstances.

The causes of institutional neurosis are environmental. There is loss of contact with the world outside the hospital or institution, and a lack of adequate occupation; this causes enforced idleness and lack of responsibility. An authoritarian hierarchical regime with an inflexible daily programme organised for the convenience of staff rather than patients increased the damaging effects of the total institution. Loss of those possessions and events (such as birthdays) that make a person an individual add to his loss of identity. He tends to have no personal friends or property and loss of prospects for the future compound the deficiencies of his already impoverished present.

Mind Persuasion

Such processes as brainwashing or mind persuasion have been developed more systematically over the last half century following Van der Lubbe's forced confession to burning the Reichstag building in 1933. Mental coercion was used during the Moscow Purge Trials in the late 1930s and developed further during the Korean War to extract enforced confessions from United States Marines. There is, of course, ancient precedent for such totalitarian methods to achieve conformity of behaviour following confession from many different parts of the world, for example, the witchcraft trials in 15th-17th Century

Europe, and similar practices have been used with varying degrees of efficacy, by some modern religious cults. Neurotic individuals are more likely to be victims of such activity.

An elaborate system of indoctrination is used to achieve 'conversion' and self-accusation resulting in the person becoming a submissive follower. Confession is extorted by high-lighting the feelings of guilt that are already latent inside people, and by creating continual uncertainty with loss of all anticipation of relief, and prevention of any hope for the future. The victim is kept absolutely alone, and drugs, sensory deprivation and torture have been used. The victim is trained to accept and believe his confession and that of others, and rehearses this continually. He is persuaded to bear false testimony to implicate other people. This is a form of neurosis provoked by extreme stress and when the person returns to normal conditions usually he repudiates his confession, and returns to the values he held before his imprisonment.

Compensation Neurosis

As neurotic attitudes intrude in all other areas of life, it is not surprising that they affect a person's interaction with justice and the law. Damages following injury are assessed by the judge and aim at restoration, which is, of course, often unattainable. Compensation is given for pain, for loss of a part or a function of the body, and also for loss of enjoyment. Where expectations for the future are impaired, due to limitation of physical or intellectual capacity, this is also taken into consideration. Financial damages, then, take into consideration the earning potential of the victim, the cost of treatment and any loss of interest incurred.

It has been known for a long time that the protracted processes of the law inhibit recovery; 'the sinister influence of litigation on the intellect may be traced very widely' (Gowers, 1892). There are a number of factors which determine how an individual will respond psychologically to injury. Clearly personality and the presence of disorder of personality is important. How the person perceives stress and the presence of other sources of insecurity (for example, loss of employment) will be influential. The nature of physical damage and its implications as psychological threat must also be taken into account.

Non-organic post-accident syndromes have been considered by Robitscher (1971) to fall into one of three categories, true traumatic neurosis, compensation neurosis or malingering. However, the number of different terms that have been used are very numerous; a few of these are listed in table 8.1.

Table 8.1 Some terms used for neurosis following an environmental precipitant

Accident neurosis	Justice neurosis
Traumatic neurosis	Triggered neurosis
Fright neurosis	American disease
Traumatic hysteria	Mediterranean disease
Traumatic neurasthenia	Greek disease
Compensation neurosis	Wharfies back
Compensationitis	Railway spine
Profit neurosis	Aftermath neurosis
Litigation neurosis	Disability neurosis
Unconscious malingering	Non-organic post-accident syndrome

True traumatic neurosis describes a neurotic reaction to a stressful event. This may be manifested in fear with resultant phobia, loss and consequent depression, inappropriate anxiety, and so on. A soldier was discharged from the Services as being 'permanently medically unfit' with anxiety neurosis. He claimed that this was provoked by being shouted at by a non-commissioned officer and made to climb a tropical mountain at midday. Another man had, when lifting iron girders at work, suffered damage to his penis without any loss of function. His wife claimed that she found his scarred penis aesthetically repulsive and refused him intercourse. For both these cases there was a claim for compensation, but for the latter case the disability or 'traumatic neurosis' occurred in the victim's wife rather than the victim himself.

Compensation neurosis describes the situation where the reaction is directly associated with likely compensation. It must, however, be unconscious; a form of *illness behaviour*. If it is deliberate simulation for gain, it is malingering. *Compensation neurosis* is more likely in situations where compensation can reasonably be expected and will be generous. Thus it is commoner in industrial than in road traffic accidents; and with larger rather than smaller employing organisations. It is commoner in men than women, in people of lower social class; and, for head injury, in those with lesser severity of injury and shorter duration of unconsciousness. Compensation may be seen as a type of secondary gain, which is both financial, and from the benefits of 'being ill'.

Forensic Aspects of Neurosis

There is an obvious association between asocial personality disorder (psychopathy) and delinquency, although it must be clearly stated that not all criminals are psychopathic, and not all people with asocial personality disorder become involved with crime. Those with asocial personality disorder may come into conflict with the law, but they also show other neurotic symptoms and behaviour; complaints of anxiety and depression are frequent and suicide quite common.

There is current interest amongst lawyers in the psychiatric reasons for carrying out criminal acts. This could be exemplified by a case of shop lifting. A middle aged woman felt herself to be increasingly alienated from her busy and successful husband. Her teenage children were becoming more independent, and she felt they used her as a servant and their home as an hotel. There was no shortage of money in the family, yet she stole a few pounds worth of groceries she did not really need from a supermarket. When interviewed about this she described her loneliness, her hopelessness, and the fact that she felt her action would draw her husband's attention to her state of despair. She was fully responsible for her behaviour, but it took place because of her neurotic depression. Obtaining a psychiatric history in order to report to the Court not only revealed clear reasons for her behaviour, but also demonstrated possible avenues for future treatment.

A more serious crime is arson. Some arsonists are suffering from psychotic illness or mental handicap. However, there are some who neither suffer from these conditions, nor show clear motivation for gain, revenge or political advantage from their act. They may give such inadequate explanation as carrying out the act because of boredom, or to gain the admiration of their peers, to get their own back on society, to exert some authority or even to gain sexual satisfaction. There is frequently other evidence of personality disorder in such people.

The commoner sexual deviations resulting in court proceedings frequently show neurotic distortion of sexual drive, for example, exhibitionism which occurs when the subject exposes his genitalia to another person, usually female, for his sexual gratification. He may masturbate during the act. Before deciding that the motivation is neurotic, especially for a first offence in an older man, depression or an organic state must be excluded. The subject is characteristically a solitary rather inadequate man who has difficulty maintaining himself in employment and, perhaps finds his dominant and robust wife critical of him, for example, in his failure to provide a higher standard of living. She may show her displeasure by withholding sex, as a punishment for his failures, although sometimes conjugal sexual relations are entirely satisfactory. He may repeatedly expose himself in the same public place to passing women. Usually such people are timid and there is no risk of extension to other sexual deviation or violence; such risk does exist if there is evidence of other, violent, antisocial behaviour.

Incest is not usually associated with neurotic illness (Bluglass, 1979). However, abnormality of personality is common, with such descriptions as 'violent' and 'irascible' occurring in 29%, and 'maladjusted at work' in 23% of convicted men. A previous criminal record was found in 46% of these men.

The Mental Health Act (1959) in its clauses concerned with compulsory admission and treatment is concerned with mental illness, psychopathic disorder, subnormality and severe subnormality as diagnostic categories. Although mental illness is not precisely defined it is normally taken to refer predominantly to psychotic disorder. However on occasions it has been used to include the severer forms of neurosis, such as hysteria with dissociation symptoms.

The Social Phenomenon of Self-poisoning

For over 70% of completed suicides, evidence of depression at the time of death can be found; type of depression cannot be specified retrospectively (Barraclough *et al.*, 1974). There is a markedly increased suicide rate for neurosis; about six times the expected rate for the normal population. Increased risk of suicide is also associated with alcoholism and drug addiction, personality disorder, especially of asocial type, and with serious physical illness.

There are two distinct but overlapping groups of people; 'suicides' who are older and more likely to be male, and 'attempted suicides' who are younger and more likely to be female. Recently the term *parasuicide* has been used to describe any individual who deliberately initiates an act of non-fatal self-injury or who ingests a substance in excess of any prescribed or generally recognised dose. Whilst the number of suicides in England and Wales has dropped by almost a third since 1960, the number of parasuicides admitted to hospital for poisoning by taking an overdose has increased more than five times; the *overdose epidemic*. Parasuicide occurs especially commonly in the second and third decades of life. It has become especially common in females from the age of 15 to 25.

The state of mind of those harming themselves is very variable, often the behaviour is impulsive and unpremeditated. Overdose is frequently an appeal for help for solutions to complicated life problems. *Attempted suicide* is a misnomer as many taking overdoses do not intend to die but rather to change their life situation. For this reason the term self-poisoning has been preferred.

Ambivalence is characteristic of the self-poisoning episode; the patient carries out an act which risks death, and at the same time uses it to further her plans and subsequent relationships in life. She both wants to die and at the same time witness the remorse of those she feels have done her an injustice. She prepares for death but at the same time, through her behaviour, makes plans for her future alive. This ambivalence may be expressed in words, but almost always in the actions of the person taking the overdose. She carries out the dangerous behaviour but at the same time tries to arrange that circumstances will probably result in her being discovered in time. For this reason, completed suicides may have been partly accidental, but have involved reckless risk-taking.

The characteristics of parasuicide have been studied in considerable detail in Edinburgh. In the 1970s there was a considerable increase in self-poisoning by late teenage girls (Kreitman and Schreiber, 1979). Parasuicide was particularly common in young women in a 'marginal' marital status, that is those who were divorced, living apart, or cohabiting with someone to whom they were not married. Teeenage married girls showed a sharper increase in para-suicide than the unmarried, and this was often associated with being the victim of violence or being in debt.

Recent consumption of alcohol is common before overdose and it is likely that this and the association with established alcohol dependence before overdose is increasing. Psychiatric diagnosis amongst parasuicides is not very reliable but, where diagnosis has been made, neuroses, especially depressive neurosis and person-ality disorder, are commonest. Parasuicide occurs in all sorts of settings although it is particularly concentrated in the poorest and most overcrowded parts of the inner city and large council housing estates. These are, of course, areas of high living stress with other social problems and a high crime rate.

A recent upsetting event is commonly described by parasuicides when interviewed soon after the event. The commonest happening to precipitate overdose is serious argument with the person regarded as being closest; husband, mother, boy friend. Arguments with other relatives, and problems at work or with finance are also common, as are feelings of depression or loneliness. Situational crisis or adverse life events in the preceding month are commonly associated with attempted suicide.

The neurotic elements of attempted (but unsuccessful) suicide are demonstrated in that it cannot be an appropriate way of dealing with stress; marital and family difficulties are often found to be associated with this behaviour. For example, there is a relationship between parasuicide and child abuse. In nearly a third of families con-taining abused or at-risk children one or both parents had attempted suicide. Both overdose and child abuse are frequent manifestations of marital difficulties often in people with underlying personality problems.

About one seventh of all acute medical admissions are for self-poisoning in Britain. In 1968 there was a recommendation by the Department of Health that all such patients should be referred to poisoning treatment centres in district general hospitals and seen by psychiatrists. It has been shown that junior doctors, nurses and social workers with suitable training and supervision by a psychiatrist can carry out the intitial assessment of overdose patients, and a psychiatric opinion is probably only required for about one in five (Leading article, 1979). More research is required into the best method of following up these patients in order to reduce subsequent self-poisoning and also into ways of preventing this disorder from occurring. The best way of treating the epidemic is by prevention.

There are valid reasons for designating neurosis as illness. It is also a social condition. It may be precipitated by social and environmental factors. Its symptomatology is quite clearly social in that it manifests in disturbed relationships. Various forms of neurotic disturbance are culture bound; particular social situations provoke specific types of neurotic reaction. Treatment of neurosis will never be efficacious unless the social milieu – family, cultural background, work conditions and nationality – are fully taken into account.

Bibliography

Asher, R. (1951). Munchausen's syndrome. *Lancet*, 1, 339–340

Bancroft, J., Skrimshire, A., Casson, J., Harvard-Watts, O. and Reynolds, F. (1977). People who deliberately poison or injure themselves: their problems and their contacts with helping agencies. *Psychol. Med.*, 7, 289–303

Barraclough, B.M., Bunch, J., Nelson, B. and Sainsbury, P. (1974). A hundred cases of suicide: Clinical aspects. *Br. J. Psychiat.*, 125, 355–373

Barton, R. (1976). *Institutional Neurosis*, 3rd edn, J. Wright & Sons, Bristol

Bluglass, R.S. (1979). Incest. *Br. J. Hosp. Med.*, 22, 152–157

Brierley, H. (1979). *Transvestism: A Handbook with Case Studies for Psychologists, Psychiatrists and Counsellors*, Pergamon Press, Oxford

Cohn, N. (1957). *The Pursuit of the Millenium*, Secker & Warburg, London

Cox, T. (1978). *Stress*, Macmillan, London

Davies, P. (1979). Motivation, responsibility and sickness in the psychiatric treatment of alcoholism. *Br. J. Psychiat.*, 134, 449–458

Department of Health and Social Security (1980). *Inequalities in Health*, H.M.S.O., London

Dominian, J. (1980). *Marital Pathology: An Introduction for Doctors, Counsellors and Clergy*, Darton & B.M.A., London

Dostoievsky, F. (1866). *The Gambler*, translated by Coulson, J., Penguin Books, Harmondsworth

Eisenberg, P. and Lazarsfeld, P.F. (1938). The psychological effects of unemployment. *Psychol. Bull.*, 35, 358–90

Fagin, L. (1981). *Unemployment and Health in Families*, DHSS, London

Fanning, D.M. (1967). Families in flats. *Br. med. J.*, 18, 382–386

Farmer, R. and Hirsch, S. (1979). *The Suicide Syndrome*, Croom Helm, London

Glatt, M.M. (1974). Alcoholism. *Br. J. Hosp. Med.*, 11, 111–120

Goffman, E. (1961). *Asylums*, Penguin Books, Harmondsworth

Gowers, W.R. (1892). *A Manual of Diseases of the Nervous System I and II*, J. & A. Churchill, London

Hagnell, O. and Kreitman, N. (1974). Mental illness in married pairs in a total population. *Br. J. Psychiat.*, 125, 293–302

Henderson, S. and Duncan-Jones, P. (1978). The patient's primary group. *Br. J. Psychiat.*, 132, 74–86

Holmes. T.H. and Rahe, R.H. (1967). The social readjustment rating scale. *J. Psychosom. Res.*, 11, 213–218

Home Office (1979). *Marriage Matters. A Consultative Document by the Working Party on Marriage Guidance*, HMSO, London

Kessel, W.I.N. (1965). Self poisoning. *Br. med. J.*, 2, 1265

Kiev, A. (1972). *Transcultural Psychiatry*, Penguin Books, Harmondsworth

Kinston, W. and Rosser, R. (1974). Disaster: Effects of mental state and physical state. *J. Psychosom. Res.*, 18, 437–456

Kreitman, N., Collins, J., Nelson, B. and Troop, J. (1970). Neurosis and marital interaction. *Br. J. Psychiat.*, 117, 33–58

Kreitman, N. and Schreiber, M. (1979). Parasuicide in young Edinburgh women 1968–75. *Psychol. Med.*, 9, 469–480

Leading Article (1979). Policies on self-poisoning. *Br. med. J.*, 2, 1091–2

Lindegard, B. (1980). *Common Mental Disorders: Epidemiological Studies on Middle-aged People in Gothenburg, Sweden*, Socialmedicinsk Information, Goteborg

Moore, N.C. (1974). Psychiatric illness and living in flats. *Br. J. Psychiat.*, 125, 500–507

Moran, E. (1975). Pathological gambling. In: *Contemporary Psychiatry* (Ed. Silverstone, T. and Barraclough, B.) Headley Brothers Ltd. Ashford, Kent

Moss, P.D. and McEvedy, C.P. (1966). An epidemic of overbreathing among schoolgirls. *Br. med. J.*, 2, 1295–1300

Oppenheimer, E., Stimson, G.V. and Thorley, A. (1979). Seven-year follow-up of heroin addicts: abstinence and continued use compared. *Br. med. J.*, 2, 627–629

Paton, A. and Saunders, J.G. (1981). ABC of alcohol. *Br. med. J.*, 283, 1248–1250

Rees, W.L. (1981). Medical aspects of unemployment. *Br. med. J.*, 283, 1630–1631

Robitscher, J. (1971). *Compensation in Psychiatric Disability and Rehabilitation*, Thomas, Springfield, Ill.

Ryle, A. (1967). *Neurosis in the Ordinary Family*, Tavistock Publications, London

Salmons, P.H. and Sims, A.C.P. (1981). Smoking profiles of patients admitted for neurosis. *Br. J. Psychiat.*, 139, 43–46

Scott, P.D. (1964). Definition, classification, prognosis and treatment. In: *The Pathology and Treatment of Sexual Deviation* (Ed. Rosen, I.), Oxford University Press, London

Shepherd, D.M. and Barraclough, B.M. (1980). Work and suicide: an empirical investigation. *Br. J. Psychiat.*, 136, 469–478

Sims, A.C.P. (1975). Dependence on alcohol and drugs following treatment for neurosis. *Br. J. Addiction*, 70, 33–40

Sims, A.C.P. (1982). Mental Illness and Urban Disaster (awaiting publication)

Sims, A.C.P., White, A.C. and Murphy, T. (1979). Aftermath neurosis: Psychological sequelae of the Birmingham bombings in victims not seriously injured. *Med. Sci. Law*, 19, 78–81

Smith, S.M., Hanson, R. and Noble, S. (1973). Parents of battered babies: a controlled study. *Br. med. J.*, iv, 388–391

St. Clare, William (1787). Country news. *The Gentleman's Magazine*, 57, 1, 268 (cited by Hunter and Macalpine 1963)

Tyhurst, J.S. (1951). Individual reactions to community disaster. *Am. J. Psychiat.*, 107, 764

Wakeling, A. (1979). A general psychiatric approach to sexual deviation. In: *Sexual Deviation*, 2nd edn (Ed. Rosen, I.), Oxford University Press

9 The Elderly Neurotic

Crabbed age and youth cannot live together;
Youth is full of pleasure, age is full of care;
Youth like summer morn, age like winter weather;
Youth like summer brave, age like winter bare;
Youth is full of sport, age's breath is short;
Youth is nimble, age is lame;
Youth is hot and bold, age is weak and cold;
Youth is wild and age is tame;
Age, I do abhor thee, youth, I do adore thee;

William Shakespeare: The Passionate Pilgrim

Much is unpredictable in our society, but one thing that is certain is that the proportion of the population which is old will undoubtedly increase. Between 1970 and 1980, the population of those aged over 65 increased by nearly one quarter. In England and Wales there were less than one and a half million people aged over 65 in 1901, about six and a half million in 1971, and expected to be seven and a half million by 1991. The number of people in England and Wales aged over 80 is expected to rise to more than 1 600 000 people by the end of the century.

An unobstrusive yet profoundly beneficial advance in medicine in the last 20 years has been the application of psychiatric diagnosis to the elderly. Whereas previously all mental disorders in old people were regarded with pessimism, it is now realised that a large number of people have treatable conditions, that the natural history of these illnesses is similar to the same conditions occurring in younger people, and that the prognosis in old age may be no worse and in some cases better than in younger people. With depression in the elderly we are faced with the same diagnostic decision that occurs in younger people: there is a group of people with biological symptoms, such as loss of appetite and weight, mental retardation, and less in the way of psychosocial precipitants who respond well to chemical treatment; there is another group of people whose precipitants appear to be more environmental and psychogenic, and understandably these people require an approach that deals with these problems rather than medication. By recognising a neurotic condition in old age, we have already made a start in helping the patient to deal with it.

Neurosis is quite common in old age (perhaps Shakespeare's 'crabbed age'); however in the past treatment for neurotic disorders was given only to younger patients (figure 9.1). In a community survey in Newcastle about 12.5% suffered from neurosis or personality disorder of

moderate severity. As in younger people, women with neurosis out-
number men. Neurosis is probably a little less common in the elderly
but as described earlier, the problem comes in deciding what is and
what is not neurosis. Very few of the elderly neurotics are referred to
hospital specifically for neurotic symptoms; quite a number of them
are however known to their general practitioners. The frequency of
neurosis in general practice varies between 10 and 20% of the elderly
population. Probably 60% of elderly neurotics are not recognised as
such, and Bergmann (1971) considers that neuroses amongst the elderly
are often inappropriately dealt with. The relatives tend to see symptoms as either an integral part of the ageing process or alternatively
an accentuation of the old person's previous character.

There are two main reasons for the increased number of elderly
neurotics. First, more neurotics now grow old and carry their neurotic
traits into old age with them (chronic neurosis). Second, there are
more people now living to a greater age, and therefore experiencing
the psychologically traumatic factors of growing old in our society
(late onset neurosis). It is the aim of this chapter to point out that
there are definite features of neurotic disturbance which may be
recognised as such and, therefore, dealt with appropriately to the
benefit of the individual. It is the intention to demonstrate that these
neurotic symptoms are not an integral part of the process of ageing.

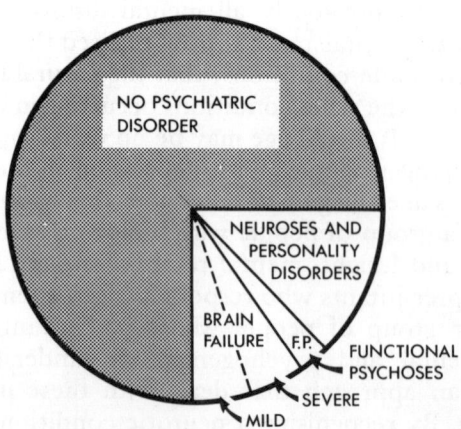

Figure 9.1   Approximate prevalence of psychiatric disorder in the general population aged 65 years

They are not a necessary complication of degenerative brain disease in an organic sense, but they are psychological reactions to stress, and therefore, avoidable or treatable in some cases.

Late Onset and Chronic Neurosis in Old Age

Approximately half the neurotic elderly population show late onset, and half chronic neurosis, although obviously there is considerable overlap. The chronic neurotic will have shown earlier in life the features described in previous chapters, that is long lasting difficulties in human relationships with resulting social isolation and poor adjustment to his current situation. The most characteristic symptom of neurosis in the elderly is hypochondriasis. There is fear of somatic symptoms, of what these predict for the future in terms of pain, serious illness and death. A woman had tyrannised her daughters throughout their life, occasionally resorting to anxiety and phobic symptoms and 'sick headaches' that proved a useful escape from unpleasant responsibilities. As she grew old she moved round each of her daughters' homes in turn, upsetting the sons-in-law, annoying her grandchildren, and worrying her daughters with her endless catalogue of complaints. Helping the family implied gently, but firmly and repeatedly pointing out to the old lady the consequences of her actions.

Late onset neurosis occurs following the stressful events of old age, especially physical illness, loneliness and the problems experienced by an isolated, physically debilitated person trying to look after herself. About 30% of physically ill elderly people have a concurrent neurotic reaction; there is almost invariably some degree of depression of mood. This figure is fairly similar to that found for depressive reaction secondary to serious physical illness in younger people. Cardiac disease is particularly likely to be associated with neurosis, which compounds the symptoms and makes diagnosis of the condition more difficult; neurosis also hinders recovery and rehabilitation. Characteristic of this was an elderly widower with cardiac asthma who was admitted to hospital following an overdose. He said he did not like to trouble his only relative, his daughter, who worked as a general practitioner. He felt his life 'had closed in on him like a tight box that stopped him breathing'. Treatment consisted of medical management to improve his respiratory function, antidepressant drugs, work with him and his daughter to help them see how they were mutually dependent, encouraging him to extend his interests, and reassuring and congratulating him as he made progress in establishing a new life style. His daughter also required help to establish an independent life, and not to feel guilty for doing some things on her own.

When the difference between neurotic old people and normal elderly community residents was investigated, late onset neurosis was present in 11% of the population aged over 65 in the community (Bergmann, 1971). Such people suffered from loneliness, and had difficulty in caring for themselves. They had few hobbies and interests. There is a strong association between physical disability and neurosis, and elderly neurotics have a high mortality rate. Hundred per cent of males and 48% of females with late onset neurosis showed some physical disability compared with only 22% of normal elderly males and 18% of females. Four years later 57% of the neurotic males and 50% of neurotic females had died: this compared with death in only 22% normal elderly males and 16% females. From life expectancy tables, twice as many neurotic males had died as expected. In another study it was shown that the level of intelligence for elderly female neurotics was lower than that expected for a normal population (Nunn *et al.*, 1974).

Patterns of Neuroses in Late Life

Pure anxiety neurosis is extremely rare in the elderly. Anxiety is usually mixed with depression, hypochondriasis and agitation. Similarly, primary hysterical neuroses do not occur in old age, and hysterical symptoms herald organic cerebral impairment, a concealed depressive illness or occasionally other physical illness, for example, carcinoma.

First occurrence of phobic states are rare, and fear of going outside, for example, is more likely to be associated with poor health and a genuinely unsatisfactory environment such as exists in the disorganised inner city areas where a high proportion of old people live. Acute obsessional neurosis is uncommon in old age. However, many disorders have an obsessional colouring, and affective disorders particularly may show a mixture of obsessional and depressive ruminations. Depressive neurosis is particularly associated with various losses. Neurasthenia occurs in those as they grow old who have been similarly afflicted through life. Long standing neurosis is particularly associated with anxiety and hypochondriasis.

Depression in the Elderly

The quotation with which this chapter starts suggests that misery is the normal state of old people. It is known that affective disorders are common in the elderly, and that they have a similar prognosis to depression in younger people. It is common for organic disorders of the brain and affective disorders to occur together in old age, but so is uncomplicated depressive illness. The frequency of depression in the population aged over 65 is about 14 per 1000 people for established manic-depressive disorder, and about 90 per 1000 for neurotic depression; that is more than 4/5 of affective disorders in the elderly are neurotic in their nature. However Post (1972) has pointed out the extreme difficulty of separating elderly depression into neurotic and psychotic categories.

Depression has been categorised into understandable misery, neurotic depression or psychotic depression (Trethowan, 1975). The distinction between understandable misery and neurotic depression is based upon the appropriateness of the response to outside stress, and its capacity for resolution with time. It would be unnatural for a wife not to grieve following her husband's death, but when this grieving persists for 10 years and totally interferes with her relationships and in carrying out her everyday life, it has transcended a normal reaction to bereavement. As in neurotic depression in younger people predisposition is a most important determinant.

Two types of personality are particularly associated with the development of depression in old age; the anankastic personality with features of insecurity and rigidity, and the affective personality who is particularly anxiety prone. Females are more likely to develop an affective disorder of neurotic type than males. Stressors are important in provoking depression in those already predisposed. Poverty alone is not an important stressor and does not account for a higher incidence of depression. The experience of loss is of course significant, whether this is through bereavement or loss of status and self-esteem and the changes of self-image that occur in old age. Coupled with loss is the effect of loneliness and this is closely linked with psychological and physical ill-health. A lame or ill old person cannot meet her friends easily; a retarded depressed person has not the will or energy to want to meet them.

Depression may be provoked by medical intervention. It is not uncommon for old people with multiple pathology to be swallowing 10 different drugs each day, and some of these may cause depression, for example, methyl dopa. Similarly, reactive depression may result from the feelings of incompetence secondary to excessive sedation from phenothiazine or benzodiazepine drugs. Nitrazepam may sedate old people with impaired metabolism, for more than 24 hours. Not uncommonly the patient's complaint of weakness may be considered depressive in origin whereas it is in fact the effect of electrolyte imbalance, perhaps hypokalaemia (potassium deficiency) secondary to the administration of a diuretic.

Experience of Loss

Old age is the time of loss and the onset of depression often follows loss. The people who have shared his life, the roles and tasks in which he has been active, and his property and status are gradually divested, and eventually life itself is lost. Whether this is a gloomy prospect or accepted with equanimity depends upon what the person believes will follow his death. What to a person without religious belief is a catastrophic accumulation of losses is seen quite differently by many believers. Bereavement is the supreme loss; most often this is a widow who battles on her own after her husband's death. How the individual sees the meaning of life and hopes for the future affects his attitude to bereavement.

Retirement may give time for interests that have long been dormant, but for which the person has previously been too busy. Alternatively, retirement may precipitate an emotional reaction in which there is felt to be loss of all that made life significant. Health, both mental and physical, is vitally important and its gradual deterioration may provoke feelings of loss; of physical function, of intellectual capacity, and fears of loss of sanity.

There is a change of self-image as the body ages, which may be extremely traumatic. A woman who had always used her good looks to get her own way became increasingly frightened as she grew older. She hated living in a cul de sac where she never met anyone. At the same time she was afraid to go out and see people because she no longer felt attractive, and she had lost all confidence in her prowess as a person. Loss of hope in the future is the final straw which renders loss of self-esteem final and catastrophic.

Psychosocial Deprivation

The effects of life crises in old age are often made worse by the victim reacting in a neurotic way to the calamity. Social factors associated with mental illness in the elderly are interrelated and cumulative. Old people are resilient in the face of severe social deprivation; the losses of old age in family, occupation, friends, income and health show little correlation with neurosis. Four-fifths of old people weather these storms of life without developing neurosis. Lower socio-economic status is associated with more mental illness in the elderly. Being married, rather than single, widowed or divorced, protects from mental illness. Those living on their own have less social support and are more likely to require admission. Community disintegration is associated with an increase in mental illness; old people are more likely to remain in disintegrating rural communities — a village in which the school and the public house has closed and half the homes are unoccupied — or disorganised city centre areas, whence the younger people have gone. Isolation is damaging; this may occur where there is a one-generation society of old people, for example, in some South Coast towns, and in old people's homes. Institutionalisation promotes the development of neurotic disorder in old people; perhaps also those who are more dependent graduate to institution earlier than those who are psychologically more robust.

Psychological and social adversity occur together. Physical illness of the patient, or death of a relative, has both psychological and social consequences. A man with a well paid job retires; there is loss of status and income. When the family grows up a woman feels nobody needs her, and she may feel useless, lonely and bored. One fifth of males and half of females aged over 65 are widowed with consequent grief and loneliness. For the widow there are often changes in living arrangements, loss of income, and loss of her role in the community. These do not necessarily cause psychological symptoms but they are powerful stresses to those who are vulnerable.

Mental illnesses (neuroses and other conditions) not only result from social isolation; they also cause it. Other people are reluctant to visit the person who has become odd, and the sufferer ceases involving himself in his usual social life. This spiral of disability is shown in table 9.1. An ill person becomes isolated and, if there is depression as well, serious alienation from other people follows. Blindness, deafness and lameness tend to make a person feel isolated. Memory loss decreases a person's ability to maintain social relationships. 'Feeling old' is inversely related to feelings of health; a person who feels he has no useful contribution is more likely to show neurotic problems of adjustment.

Table 9.1   *Mental Illness in Old Age: A Factor of Escalating Psychosocial Deprivation*

Social Isolation	Mental Illness
Loss of Contact with Reality	Disorientation
Loss of affectional bonds	Memory loss
Persecutory ideas	Irritability
Neglect of helping agencies	Loss of Intellectual Grasp
	Irrational Fears
	Neglect of appearance

Problems with Relationships

Attitudes in human relationships become more rigid in old age; people may be approved whole-heartedly, or disliked quite intolerantly. An inadequate daughter who had been regarded as stupid all her life, was treated with even greater disdain by her ageing father. As she was the only person he regularly talked to, he became disgruntled through loneliness.

New stresses may occur in marriage for the elderly. Retirement of the husband may result in his wife's complaint that 'he is under my feet all the time', whilst he may express his frustration and boredom in irritability towards his wife. Physical illness of one partner may make demands of the healthy spouse which may become a considerable strain. The diminution of libido of one partner may create a problem for the other wishing to continue a more active sex life. Remarriage of the elderly is becoming more common, and sometimes there are problems in adaptation. Where the previous marriage was unsatisfactory, only too often the new partner has similar attributes of personality. Alternatively, a very different spouse may be chosen, and the person may find himself unable to adjust to the new way of life required of him, both in the social and sexual sphere.

Other family relationships may become stressful in old age. The parent used to an authoritarian role towards his children may find himself a guest in their homes without, in his eyes, any rights or personal territory. There are frequently stresses in households where three generations live together. The old person disapproves of the behaviour and the manner of upbringing of the grandchildren, who in their turn, find the grandparent rigid, intolerant and demanding.

Those living in Old People's Homes or other institutions may fail to adjust because of difficulties with relationships. This depends on their personality and attitude towards the institution, which they may see as either an oppressive prison, a shameful end in the workhouse or, alternatively, a well deserved home shared with like-minded old people. The neurotic person living in an institution, as one might expect, shows considerably more problems in adjustment than others. He suffers more from isolation and loneliness and has more difficulties with relationships.

Work and Retirement

There has grown up a myth that retirement is necessarily associated with psychological disturbance. There is in fact no proven association between retirement and suicide or increased likelihood of admission for psychiatric illness, increased rate of referral to a psychiatrist, or symptoms of emotional disturbance presenting to the general practitioner. Retirement itself does not have deleterious effects on health. It is the mental attitude towards retirement which is important; it may be met with resignation, denial or acceptance. A few months before his reluctant retirement a man said: 'What a waste of my skills to retire just now'. He spent the three years of retirement before his death in bad-tempered idleness. Preparation should be made for retirement with plans for activity and cooperation from relatives. Neurosis (of late onset) is much more likely to occur in a person who retires without preparation, with no hobbies or interests, with few friends outside work, and who then develops a physical illness. Pre-retirement courses arranged for employees are helpful, but so often it is those who will retire successfully who elect to attend.

Such problems of adjustment as boredom, feeling useless, and worries about money follow retirement. Clearly a person with no interests outside his work, or somebody who bolsters his lack of confidence with his status at work is at a considerable disadvantage. The neurotically predisposed has more problems of this sort. The only glimmer of hope that could encourage a man aged 67 who had both severe emphysema and depression was the thought of returning to his unpaid job as a guide around a medieval cathedral. Here, he found peace, interest and status.

Personality and Personality Disorder

Previous personality is an important consideration in neurosis of old age, especially chronic neurosis. As people age they become less flexible, less tolerant of ambiguity, and more resistant to change. 'It comes hard to break the habits of a lifetime.' They are more cautious and tend to accept the environment passively. There is less emphasis on achievement and more on ethical issues. There is greater preoccupation with self, and a feeling of loss of the ability to control events. Having described this stereotype there are, of course, many exceptions.

Rigid, insecure and over-anxious personalities are particularly prone to neurotic disturbance. Personality characteristics of such people are accentuated in old age. Rigidity becomes intolerance, insecurity crippling self-doubt, and proneness to anxiety may result in paralysing over-conscientiousness. A middle-aged woman consulted her doctor with depression, anxiety and guilt. It turned out that these were provoked by her elderly father who lived with the family. He was consumed with anxiety over whether he was a nuisance and was forever apologising for being in the house. This exasperated his daughter. Helping her entailed treating the old man for his anxiety and encouraging him to take a more positive attitude to helping his daughter in the home. She had to be persuaded to allow him to be helpful.

Suspicious, solitary people often make a good adjustment to old age as long as they are in good health and can remain independent. Although isolated and sometimes regarded as eccentric, they do not complain of loneliness. Similarly, passive, dependent people who may have had problems arising at work from their personality, in old age accept living in an institution or dependence upon younger relations with equanimity.

The aggressive, sociopathic personality is less likely to be physically aggressive or collide with the law in old age. However, such people may destroy personal relationships and become the nucleus for arguments in an old people's home or living with younger relations. They may dominate those around them by unpredictable gestures of hostility or self-violence. An old man used to sit near the front door of an old people's home glowering and using his walking stick to trip up the unwary; when successful he would smile slyly as he terrorised the other residents. There was no treatment except to try and occupy him elsewhere.

Those people with very low self-esteem remain miserable, adapting poorly to the dependence following bad health. The histrionic manipulative person when old, remains destructive in personal relationships perhaps controlling the behaviour of the whole family from her strategically placed sick-bed.

Alcoholism and Drug Dependence

Two sorts of alcohol problem present in the elderly — persistently heavy drinkers who continue to drink to excess, and moderate drinkers whose drinking only becomes excessive in late life (Glatt *et al.*, 1978). The two main causative factors are personality, especially anxiety prone personalities, and social, particularly the response to bereavement or retirement with consequent boredom and loneliness. Alcohol problems of the elderly occur more in females than males; they may occur in extreme old age. The most likely drugs on which there is dependence in old age are those prescribed by doctors for sedation; barbiturates were especially likely to result in addiction and there are many people at least emotionally dependent upon benzodiazepines.

Because situational problems have so often provoked an alcoholic reaction, treatment will necessitate investigating the social state and taking steps to help, for example, with housing problems or isolation. Measures to give the old person a feeling of self-respect by enabling him to be useful are highly beneficial. Complete abstinence is not necessarily an essential of treatment for the elderly alcoholic; similarly when there is a degree of dependence upon prescribed drugs it is important to weigh the discomfort and social inconvenience of withdrawal against its potential benefits.

Treatment for the Elderly Neurotic

Some aspects of treatment are different for the elderly from other neurotic patients. A type of psychotherapy needs to be practised which includes, as specific objectives of therapy: coping with death, physical ill-health and hypochondriasis, the problem of dependency and the rather different set of interpersonal relationships which is characteristic of old age (Bergmann, 1978). Hope is of great value in combating feelings of loss, but it cannot be grafted onto a background of total disbelief. The therapist should recruit the elderly person's own faith where this exists, and help him to work out how this can be applied in his present situation. Quite often a person who has suppressed his religious feelings during the busy middle of life allows himself to reflect in old age, and works out what his beliefs mean to him. Far from being neurotic, this is evidence of personal growth.

Treatment of neurosis is quite unlike many other forms of medical treatment. Making the diagnosis does not automatically lead to the prescription of this drug, or carrying out that operation. Treatment requires exploring the antecedents and seeing what can be done to reverse them, helping the patient to see how he got into this situation and staying with him until he finds a way out, working with him and his family to resuscitate mangled relationships and unravel longstanding misunderstandings. There is no simple formula for this sort of treatment; what can be recommended is to investigate the history without becoming involved in the drama. Sometimes there is no solution.

For chronic neurosis, insight as to how the patient affects others, and reassurance that symptoms do not signify physical illness, is helpful. Late onset neurosis often responds to more active treatment; psychotherapy is not restricted to young patients. It can be very helpful for the elderly when the goals of treatment are clearly recognised. The aim is to help the patient adjust to losses and the threats of loss. The resources for achieving this aim belong to the patient and it is the task of psychotherapy to make what he already has available

to him. Lengthy analysis to explore childhood conflicts is not indicated but helping the person to have some understanding as to how
he reached this state of misery, how he impinges on other people,
and how he can start to reverse this process is valuable.

Coming to terms with the loss of those close to him through bereavement requires genuine sympathy from those around during acute
grief in facing reality and bearing pain, and then support in taking up
the normal routine of daily life again. Grief is unpleasant but necessary, and numbing the patient with sedative drugs may be counter-
productive; drugs are not normally indicated. As well as bereavement,
the old person has to come to terms with his own physical weakness
and anticipation of death. Coping with these concerns will draw
upon the patient's resources in terms of his beliefs about life and
death and his relationship with family and friends.

There is an enormous variety of different community and residential
services for the elderly — both statutary and voluntary (Gray and
Isaacs, 1979). Social services for the elderly should allow people to
do as much for themselves as possible. Pre-retirement courses are useful; the recently retired often find occupation and fulfilment in
helping others — organising voluntary services for other old people,
helping those older and more infirm than themselves, looking after
grandchildren whilst parents are at work and so on. Providing ready-
made social organisations for old people is fraught with difficulty
and it is best, where possible, to give support to organisations that
already exist, for example, arranging transport for an infirm old
person to reach her Senior Citizen's club or weekly bingo night.
There is a great need for day centres of various types; places where
old people can go and do things, or at least watch others doing things
— and socialise as little or as much as they like.

Perhaps the single most important part of treatment for the elderly
neurotic is the fostering of independence and self-care. There are so
many pressures to remove independence from the very old person,
especially if physically or mentally ill, and there is some evidence to
suggest that once having been made dependent by meeting all social
needs, it is very difficult and unlikely for the neurotic to re-establish
a pattern of self-reliance. This further diminishes self-esteem. It is
very much better to provide aids to retain independence than to
institutionalise, even if the former entails more expense for the public
organisation and more effort from the helper.

Summary

In this chapter we have discussed the elderly neurotic. We have described the psychological, social and physical events which are common to all old people, and we have discussed how a small proportion of people react to these by showing neurotic symptoms. Although only the minority are neurotic, as the total number of old people grows greater into the next century, so the amount of neurotic disability in old age will also increase.

We have discussed late onset neurosis in which there is a neurotic reaction to features in the environment related to growing old, and chronic neurosis, that is the situation when a neurotic person grows old. Most of the different types of neurosis described in earlier chapters also occur in the elderly, especially depression and hypochondriasis. The distinctive patterns of personality disorder and also of alcholism in the elderly have been described. We have also discussed attitudes towards retirement, the changing nature of relationships in old age and the experience of loss.

Treatment for neurosis in the elderly is based upon maintaining social involvement but at the same time avoiding unnecessary dependence upon others. The importance of the person's own beliefs, especially about death, has been stressed. The skilled helper uses the patient's own resources in treatment. Neurosis relating to loneliness and physical illness can often be treated effectively by attention to the patient's individual needs.

Bibliography

Bergmann, K. (1971). The neuroses of old age. In: *Recent Developments in Psychogeriatrics* (Ed. Kay, D.W.K. and Walk, A.), Headley Brothers, Ashford, Kent

Bergmann, K. (1978). Neurosis and personality disorder. In: *Studies in Geriatric Psychiatry* (Ed. Isaacs, A.D. and Post, F.), John Wiley, New York

Busse, E.W. and Pfeiffer, E. (1973). *Mental Illness in Later Life*, American Psychiatric Association, Washington, D.C.

Gray, B. and Isaacs, B.(1979). *Care of the Elderly Mentally Infirm*, Tavistock Publications, London

Glatt, M.M., Rosin, A.M. and Jauhar, P. (1978). Alcoholic problems in the elderly. *Age and Ageing*, 7, Suppl., 64-66

Nunn, C., Bergman, K., Britton, P.G., Foster, E.M., Hall, E.H. and Kay, D.W.K. (1974). Intelligence and neurosis in old age. *Br. J. Psychiat.*, 124, 446-52

Post, F. (1972). The management and nature of depressive illness in later life: A follow-up study. *Br. J. Psychiat.*, 121, 393-404

Trethowan, W.H. (1975). Pills for personal problems. *Br. med. J.*, 4, 749-751

10 General Principles of Treatment

> ... 'there is a relationship between cowman and cows.
> If it is a good relationship, it appears that the cows
> approved the cowman ... if the cows have confidence
> in their cowman they yield better. However, it is
> easier to show the relationship than to explain it'.
>
> M.F. Seabrook, *The Relationships*
> *between Dairy Cows and Man*

An Approach to Treatment

Too often with neurosis, description of a method of treatment has
not been accompanied by definition of the patient population or
evidence for efficacy. This and the next chapter are intended for
those who are not experienced in particular forms of treatment,
but who come into contact with neurosis in their daily work and
require some general principles. This is therefore eclectic and practical at the risk of being simplistic, and does not represent any theoretical purity. The whole discussion of treatment for neurosis
must be considered provisional. We know very little about the
efficacy of different types of treatment and until we know more
we should not be dogmatic.

I am recommending no specific school or psychotherapy, nor
teaching the reader how to practise a particular form of treatment.
I hope some readers will extract for themselves what they can best
use from the different theoretical standpoints. Busy doctors, social
workers, nurses, occupational therapists and others who see neurotic
clients or patients every day require a synopsis of the treatment
methods available, and some guidance on the commonsense of
management for their patients. Technical terms have particular
meaning for different schools of opinion, but an attempt is made
here to avoid jargon as far as possible and to concentrate upon
what is important for the non-specialist in treatment. Everyone
will come across neurosis but not all neurotics should be referred
to specialists.

The Patient's Contribution to Treatment

The gist of this book has been that the importance of neurosis
does not lie solely in the severity of symptoms, but also in how
complaints are related to their social context. This is equally true

for treatment, which necessarily involves relationships. The neurotic lives in a society in which physical symptoms are acceptable but psychological symptoms are not. He has been told frequently by the time he reaches a psychiatrist, 'Just pull yourself together'. This advice has not worked, yet when patients are followed-up, those who have improved often describe their improvement in these terms, 'I just pulled myself together'.

It seems that this is what was needed, but the patient did not know how to achieve it, and he had no expectation that it was possible, and so after so many failures, he did not feel like trying. Looking at the improvement that sometimes follows a single therapeutic interview, it was concluded that in some way, the interview conveyed to the patient that he must do something himself about his condition, and also gave him some glimmer of insight as to how he could do this.

The aim of treatment is not to tell the patient to 'pull yourself together'. This has been said to him repeatedly, and it simply serves to reinforce his hopelessness, and hence his apathy. He becomes paralysed with despair. The aim is to convey to the patient that 'it is possible to pull yourself together'. It is this hope, when apprehended by the patient, that allows him to improve, and this is the first essential of treatment. When methods of treatment diminish this belief they are damaging to the patient. It is essential for the patient to realise that he is responsible for his actions and hence, to some extent, for his environment. The neurotic paradigm suggests inevitability (chapter 5); a future course through life of immutable diminuendo.

In treatment, patterns of behaviour are shown to be comprised of separate actions, and each action is shown to be within the patient's control. Although the pattern seems to follow a predetermined, destructive course, the individual actions each represent a choice. If even a minute part of the previously remorseless pattern can be altered by some deliberate action of the patient, then he and the therapist can use this to try and effect a larger and more significant change. The message of the therapist then becomes not 'pull yourself together' but, 'you have been able to pull yourself together'. Therapeutic choices can occur; for example, a man with social and sexual problems (to everyone's surprise) made satisfactory choice of marriage partner. This freed him from an apparently inevitable pattern of unsatisfactory relationships and allowed a more general improvement in his life-situation to begin.

Active involvement of the patient in treatment is essential. With physical illness, often passive resignation only is required: In psychosis, successful treatment may take place even against the opposition of the patient, but with neurosis there can never be improvement unless the therapist and the patient share objectives. Doing something that he would not otherwise do in order to get better may be the most significant factor in initiating the change which eventually results in his improvement. Treatment must seem to the patient to be reasonable: perhaps it is the thoroughness with which 'response prevention' is carried out that recommends it as an appropriate treatment for the compulsive handwasher; physiotherapy appears appropriate to the patient in the treatment of hysterical paralysis of a limb because it is a physical treatment for a physical symptom.

The patient's involvement in his own treatment demonstrates his confidence in the therapist and his motivation for change. Without this trust and motivation, an attempt at treatment will be not only useless but perhaps even destructive. For instance, a person who takes part in group psychotherapy with no confidence in the therapist or the method of treatment and no intention to modify his attitudes or behaviour is harmful to other group members. In order for the neurotic to be motivated, he must believe in the possibility of change, that improvement can occur. This confidence is often lacking, and so the therapist must demonstrate that at least some small improvement is both possible and necessary.

Why Treat Neurosis?

Why is it important to treat neurosis? Many doctors — psychiatrists, general physicians, general practitioners — do not proceed further than diagnosis with the neuroses. As long as a serious physical illness or major psychiatric disorder has been excluded, they feel their job is completed. Neurosis should be treated because, first, it is extremely common. Of course, only those, of the many with neurotic symptoms, who request treatment should receive therapy. Second, we have discussed the serious consequences of neurosis, both for the individual and upon those around him. There is an increased mortality, marked morbidity and resulting unhappiness and social disturbance. The third reason is that people seek treatment for neurotic symptoms. They will consult doctors and related professionals whether we like it or not, and we should therefore make our management as effective as possible. It is likely that the person whom the patient chooses to consult is in a better position to recommend treatment than anyone else to whom he may refer the patient.

Very many different types of treatment have been used for neurosis, and only rarely have they been assessed for their effectiveness in any rational way. In chapter 5 we have discussed methods of evaluation of treatment. Perhaps the chief contribution that health professionals, as opposed to volunteers, well-wishers and friends, can make to the treatment of the neuroses, is in the evaluation of their treatment methods. All sorts of helping and caring agencies, voluntary bodies, charitable individuals, friendly neighbours, try to do something to ease the state of neurotics. They often become enthusiastic about their methods and propagate these. From the healthy scepticism about treatment, which is part of the medical tradition, knowledge has been gained about methods of evaluation, for example, of new drugs. The treatments of neuroses need to be carefully assessed, so that no treatment method is released onto the public without a thorough trial for efficacy and a careful search for side-effects.

Aims of Treatment

In neurosis it is difficult to define the aims of treatment, and to what extent those aims can realistically be achieved; so, there is the dilemma of how much improvement, or change in life style, or 'happiness' one is aiming at. A patient after concluding 18 months out-patient treatment, said, 'I am alright, I have lost no time from work, I am not a bundle of joy, but if I was I would think there was something the matter with me'. This statement perhaps illustrates the need to have limited but realistic goals in treatment, shared by patient and therapist.

The aims of treatment are at different levels (Marks, 1974). Few therapists would feel that just giving the patient a pleasurable experience was an adequate form of treatment. There are three discrete aims: First is the treatment of the specific symptoms, for example, relieving the patient of her phobia for cats: The second is overall improvement in the patient's state with a lessening of symptoms and improved social functioning: The third is the principle of rehabilitation, that is, optimising the patient's capacity for independent action, despite the existence of residual disability. The aim is to maintain improvement and help the person to function as well as possible although recognising that there are still limitations.

Diagnosis

Before discussing the treaters, I would like to mention three controversial issues concerned with the viewpoint of treatment in neurosis; diagnosis, terminology for the recipient of help, and science. Diagnosis is a prerequisite to rational treatment. By diagnosis, I

do not imply one word containing the whole truth; 'pneumonia'
. . . I mean a diagnostic formulation; what the problem is and how
it arose. The professional mental health worker conceptualises the
problem within his own frame of reference to enable him to discuss
this person's situation with others and to decide which of the available treatment facilities he should recruit.

Amongst psychiatric referrals, neurosis is diagnosed from functional psychosis, organic psycho-syndrome, or mental handicap.
For the general practitioner, neurotic symptoms need to be separated
from physical illness. For the social worker, neurosis must be distinguished from problems wholly ascribed to adverse social circumstances. The second stage of 'diagnosis' is to formulate the neurotic
problem in descriptive psychopathological, behavioural, psychodynamic and social terms so that the patient's condition becomes
meaningful to the therapist and he knows where to start treatment.
To explain these terms: by *descriptive psychopathological*, I mean
a precise empathic description of symptoms that shows that the
therapist understands what it is the patient experiences; *behavioural*,
implies description of the inappropriate behaviour analysed into its
component parts; *psychodynamic* how did the symptoms arise from
this individual's background experience?; *social* points out the need
to attend to the environmental context in which the problem arose.

Patients and Clients

In discussing treatment, I have consistently referred to 'patient'
rather than 'client'. This is quite deliberate, the word patient refers
to suffering, and whatever the cause treatment aims to alleviate
pain. This is the first essential for the therapist. The word client
is of more doubtful parentage. The Latin word implies servile conformity of the client to the whims of his patron; a position of
subordination. In more recent usage a client pays for services which
he demands irrespective of what might be best for him.

The word was taken into dynamic psychotherapy because clients
were not ill, and it represented the financial contract between
client and therapist. It has now come into use to refer to the recipient of attention from the social worker or counsellor. I consider
that, because of its origins, 'client' has unfortunate overtones and is
inferior to 'patient'.

Science and Medicine

The third area of controversy concerns 'science'. Medicine is not a
science; it uses and applies science. It also uses manual dexterity,

for example, in the work of a neurosurgeon. Similarly, psychiatry as a branch of medicine is not a science, but it needs to use and apply scientific knowledge, such as psychology, which is the study and understanding of human thought and behaviour.

Psychiatry should enlist any methods of treatment that are beneficial whatever their origins; scientific method should be used to evaluate efficacy. Psychiatrists require a sound basis of psychology to carry out their work. When clinical psychologists treat patients they are no longer acting as scientists; scientific purity has been subjugated to the best interests of the individual patient; this is necessarily incurred by practice. In a sense every treatment of a patient is an experiment. However, as it cannot be adequately controlled, it is also the intuitive application of an acquired craft. There is often some conflict between science, technique and the use of personal attributes in the practice of medicine.

Treatment by Whom?

There is no single route to becoming a therapist. It is a complex mixture of training and experience, attitudes and personal characteristics which determines whether the therapist will be effective or not. It is also important to consider the match between therapist and patient; how the patient sees the therapist and the nature of the communication between them.

The experience of the therapist will be at one of three levels. First, there is the intuitive level. Some people because of their own qualities seem intrinsically to be helpful in human relationships and in furthering the aspirations of other people. Such a person may be drawn into a caring profession, but without further training is likely to be naive in evaluating people's problems, over-optimistic in assessing the possibility for improvement, and blind to the complications of intervention. The second stage of experience is the result of general professional training and practice. In the past there has been very little training in the treatment of neuroses for doctors during their undergraduate medical course, and this was often deficient for social workers, nurses and others. There is generally more practical training in interviewing now, and in learning about the nature of the exchange between patient and therapist. The third level of experience is more specialist training in a method of treatment of the neuroses. This is usually gained in an intensive personal involvement of some type, for example, a personal dynamic training analysis or individual apprentice-style training from a teacher in behavioural modification, or carrying out a substantial clinical research study of neurosis and its treatment, requiring contact with patients.

In one sense the professional allegiance of the therapist-doctor, psychologist, social worker, nurse, occupational therapist — is irrelevant. His personal qualities, experiences, and preparedness to learn are much more important. However, the neurotic patient may have preconceived opinions of a certain profession which preclude his even making contact with somebody from that group, and so, in practice, the profession is important. The patient's expectations are important but difficult to evaluate as they may be influenced by his underlying neurotic conflict. As an example of one type of further specialist training in psychotherapy, one could cite the intensive practical training over 18 months undertaken by the *nurse therapist* (Bird *et al.*, 1979). This provides practical experience in behavioural modification. The nurse learns how to screen neurotic patients for suitability, carry out behavioural analysis, plan and undertake specific treatment and arrange discharge from treatment, and follow-up.

In some counselling organisations the counsellors may be professional, for example, school counsellors; in others they are volunteers. Increasingly, it is realised that people should be selected for such work, and relevant training is essential. For instance, an organisation aiming to help and befriend those who are bereaved arranges courses for prospective befrienders. Before someone is taken on as a volunteer it is ensured that sufficient time has elapsed since their own bereavement, otherwise their counselling might be more a way of resolving their own problems, rather than beneficial to the 'clients'. It would be invidious to list voluntary organisations concerned with helping neurotic people. They are generally not aimed specifically at neurosis, but simply find that a certain proportion of those with whom they deal do in fact suffer from neuroses.

Constructive help is not confined to professionals, or even trained volunteers. Neurotics who have improved often describe family, friends, people at work, their Minister, the hairdresser, etc., as having been helpful. This fact needs to be accepted and used by the professionals. How can someone become more effective in helping people? The answer to this question is in fact very complicated, but at risk of over-simplification: (1) he wants to help other people; (2) he knows enough about himself to be able to use himself as a therapeutic tool; (3) he learns how people in general interact in relationships; (4) he gets to know this specific individual who needs help; and (5) he creates an atmosphere of optimistic acceptance in which the neurotic person realises that his behaviour can change, at least slightly, in a beneficial direction and that this change is expected of him.

The characteristics of treaters have been studied in some detail. The value of such qualities as warmth, genuineness and empathy has been shown (Truax and Carkhuff, 1967). It is probable that these qualities can be learnt to some extent as well as being innate. An interesting comment on how such characteristics are beneficial in other relationships is shown by the description given by Seabrook (1973) for the qualities of the ideal cow-man in helping his non-human charges to deliver a high milk yield.

Modelling is an essential part of treatment (Bandura, 1978). Whether the therapist intends it or not he will inevitably become a model for his patient's behaviour. In their fantasies, his patients will invest him with qualities he does not have, and what he does will be watched with intense interest by the patient, and parts of his behaviour will be copied by them. This modelling is used in behavioural treatment. For example, the therapist treating a patient for compulsive handwashing will soil his own hands and so demonstrate to the patient that he comes to no harm. In a therapeutic situation in which there is close contact between the patient and therapist, especially when the therapist has an active roll, for example, the sister in charge of a Day Unit, modelling may be a most important part of therapy. It was found in such a Day Hospital that patients who talked about wishing to take up psychiatric nursing as a future career generally did well. On closer inspection, they were found to be modelling themselves on the cheerful, stable, commonsensical sister in charge of the unit. This obviously has considerable implications for the selection of staff. Their personal attributes and stability are more important than academic attainments.

Methods and Principles of Helping

The therapist must know what he is trying to achieve. He needs to formulate what would constitute improvement for this patient; relief of symptoms or lessening of destructiveness in relationships. His next aim is to achieve an appropriate level of involvement; he is concerned to help the patient, and the patient needs to be convinced that his therapist is concerned. Over-involvement of the therapist can become a crippling burden for the patient to carry; he feels that if he lets the therapist down all will be lost. This usually occurs when the patient reawakens the therapist's own neurotic conflicts. The therapist must realise this, and work through his own difficulties or alternatively, avoid patients that provoke such a reaction.

The Non-directive Approach

The theoretical difference between different types of treatment or different schools of thought, is not the most significant factor as far as the outcome of patients is concerned. However, certain philosophical stances carry implications for treatment. For example, *non-directive therapy* has become a sacred cow for some counsellors, but this idea itself contains a paradox. Clearly the aim of therapy is that some change will be effected, and the direction of this change will partly be determined by the therapist. At the same time directing the patient into a pattern of behaviour is deprecated by some on ideological grounds, and by others because in practice it has not worked.

Why is this emphasis on non-directive treatment? First, one cannot in fact change a person's pattern of behaviour by giving them good advice; other contingencies need to be built in. Second, the therapist does not know exactly what course of action would benefit his patient most, nor what the patient really wants. We should, therefore, be very cautious before directing the patient. However, by not giving his patient any clear lead, the therapist can suggest that he carries no responsibility for the outcome of treatment; this is an unjustifiable evasion.

Quite often we do know what is best for our patients, perhaps not in a specific way but in general terms. So although we could harm them by prescribing certain activities, we can also harm them by withholding our understanding of life situations. For example, we know that it is beneficial for the way a person regards himself to be in work rather than unemployed. We know that, in general, children fare better when their parents live with them at home together. We can often help our patients by directing their attention away from their own immediate problems to the more general principles involved and what is usually the most satisfactory course of action in such situations. That is, we can objectify for them, and we can comment upon the probable outcome following both a non-neurotic and a neurotically-derived decision.

Non-directiveness is itself a form of direction. For example, the non-directive therapist may encourage his patient in talking about the relationship with his parents by looking at him expectantly when this subject is mentioned, and looking out of the window when the patient talks about his symptoms. It would be a mistake to consider this to be non-directive. It is simply shaping the patient's behaviour so that non-verbal cues are used in a more sophisticated way. There can be no such thing as truly non-directive treatment.

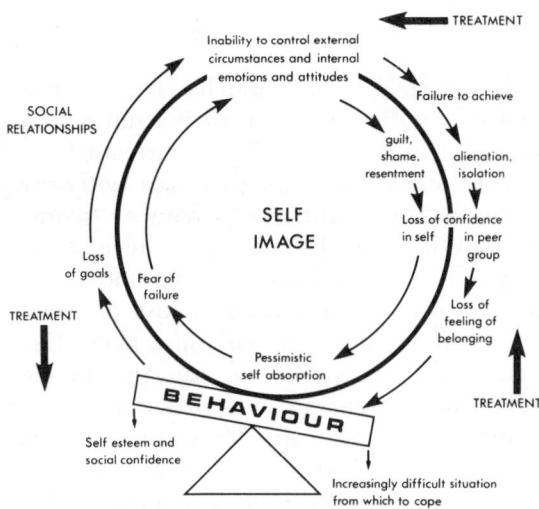

Figure 10.1   Treatment to combat dependence

Coping and Independence

Coping and achieving independence is a fundamental aim of treatment. Frank (1974) has described *demoralisation*, the state of mind when a person feels unable to cope with a problem which he, and those about him, expect him to be able to handle. It sets up a vicious circle in which there is crippling loss of self-esteem and inability to cope with relationships. This is demonstrated in figure 10.1. Loss of self-confidence occurs with an inability to master external circumstances or internal feelings. This produces a sense of failure and guilt, with shame and resentment. Feelings of alienation, and isolation result because he feels everybody else is able to cope more effectively. This leads to a loss of belief in the social group to which he belongs and a consequent loss of the feeling of belonging. Pessimistic self-absorption, loss of any goals, with fear of future failure in relationships and in the ability to control his own fears repeats the whole cycle. As this destructive process proceeds it becomes increasingly difficult to reverse it.

Treatment entails the patient learning how he can help himself. The therapist starts by demonstrating that the patient already has some achievements; for example, at least he did manage to come for treatment today, and he has managed to survive this long. Reassurance of this type, sharing the patient's minutest successes as they occur without patronising, and without dwelling on failures, is beneficial. With the patient's active cooperation attainable goals are set for the next interview, and when these result in success, discussion ensues in which a plan is made to generalise from these successes.

As treatment proceeds it is gradually suggested to the patient that the relationship with the therapist is itself a support of which he will ultimately be independent. This must not be communicated as rejection, but as the gradual and appropriate withdrawal of support such as might occur in teaching a person to swim. Initially the patient knows that he can obtain help if he loses his confidence. This accessibility of support is progressively removed.

In neurosis the sufferer experiences a loss of freedom; a loss of the capacity to control his own circumstances. He feels himself to be paralysed whilst everyone else can fly. In treatment he is helped to realise that he can in fact walk, although perhaps with a limp, and other people also can only walk, although more freely.

Successful behavioural treatment of a phobic neurosis may be effective because it demonstrates to the patient that this part of his behaviour has come under his own control to an extent that he did not think possible (Gelder, 1979). Similarly, successful psychodynamic treatment presents the patient with a theory of causation; conflicts that became unconscious following infantile psychic trauma. When the patient is convinced that there is a cause, and that he can carry out work which returns him to and deals with those early infant conflicts, he gains control once again over the course of his life. This element of handing back to the patient, who feels trapped by his own impotence to deal with externally imposed inevitability, responsibility for his present state and future progress, can be seen in many different types of treatment.

Another fundamental factor in treatment is the relationship between the helper and the sufferer. The patient expresses some degree of trust by coming for treatment. He needs to be confident both in the therapist as an individual, and in his role as demonstrated by his professional training and standing. A temporary stage of dependence during the earlier phase of treatment progresses to an alliance in which the patient begins to have some insight into the nature of his problems and their causes.

Collusion and Confrontation

A general principle of treatment for neurosis is the aim of helping the patient to gain insight and escape from his symptoms whilst avoiding both collusion and confrontation. This is well exemplified in the treatment of hysteria. It is accepted that the patient genuinely needs help. The doctor reassures her that improvement is possible but at the same time avoids collusion with her in accepting her physical explanation of aetiology. Once he is seen to be colluding his ability to treat is severely limited.

It is important for the patient to feel that she and her symptoms are accepted by the doctor as real and worthwhile treating. Patients and their relatives tend to dichotomise into physical illness, which is genuine, and 'imaginary' psychological symptoms, which are not. It is important for the doctor to show that he considers symptoms to be genuine without making any comment on their cause, thus avoiding confrontation. The therapeutic team does not try and demonstrate associations between symptoms and social or psychological difficulties but they try to understand for themselves the features of 'secondary gain' from the sick role. How does the patient benefit from being ill? A situation is then constructed where the gains from getting better outweigh the advantages of illness.

A 27-year-old housewife was admitted to hospital following two years increasing immobility; eventually she was confined to a wheel chair during the day and a couch downstairs at night. She also described episodes of unconsciousness occurring once or twice a week. As she was unable to look after her three children, her husband had arranged for a young woman to help, and she was living in the house, sleeping upstairs with the patient's husband. When the patient was admitted to hospital her husband wished to exclude her from home and live with his new mistress and the three children. He refused to have her home at weekends and changed the lock on the front door. The patient was not concerned about her husband but wanted to retain custody of the children.

She was discharged after ten weeks in hospital. She had regained full use of her legs; she had had no further attacks, she was on no medication and she was able to carry out housework adequately. She had come to realise that she was most likely to gain custody of her children by demonstrating her competence to look after them. Intensive physiotherapy had been used with graded exercises towards walking and plenty of work for her to carry out on the ward between sessions. Psychotherapy had concentrated upon her feelings towards her husband and her children, and helping her to formulate plans for the future on leaving hospital. Group discussion similarly had concentrated on the practical and solvable aspects of her family problems.

Insight and Self-control

For satisfactory adjustment or 'congruence', the patient has to find a balance between accepting the present circumstances if they cannot be changed and resolving to improve what is possible. Insight can only be achieved for himself; it cannot be forced reluctantly

or incredulously upon him. The father of a family may realise that
he has been acting the despotic king at home, or alternatively the
faceless person whose sole function is to earn money for food,
clothes and the television licence. He has to learn what conflicts
have shaped his present behaviour; perhaps his absorption with
work developed as he felt excluded by the friendship between
his wife and his son. He comes to see how this has arisen, and how
his present behaviour relates to 'the sort of person I am'. Treatment
implies taking on (1) new attitudes, and (2) a change of behaviour.
Both of these are necessary; one cannot tell which will come first
although frequently change of behaviour precedes attitudinal change.
Different types of treatment concentrate upon the patient taking
responsibility for his own actions; that is on methods of self-control.

Learning self-control involves various stages. The patient observes
and records the behaviour which needs to be changed: the number
of sleeping tablets, the frequency of hand washing. He then relates
this behaviour to other experiences of life, both to external circumstances (problems at work) and to internal experiences (feeling
tense and harried). He notes the frequency of occurrence of the
behaviour and also what measures are effective in preventing it.
When he achieves success, he allows himself some sort of reward.
These stages are very simple but the fact that the neurotic has
come for treatment means that they have failed to work for him
in the past; probably at the stage of evaluation he is too critical of
his performance and does not allow himself rewards. Treatment
may mean the therapist watching the process of self-control and
helping the patient to realise where blocks are occurring.

Developing a relationship with the therapist, learning how symptoms have developed, and learning how to control them in the
treatment situation is not enough. A vital part of treatment is for
the patient to learn to internalise, to make his own, what has been
suggested from outside. This constitutes the *homework* of, for example,
behaviour modification. A patient, phobic for spiders, controls
his symptoms by exposure to dead spiders during a treatment session.
It is then very important for him to practise this same exposure
regularly at home before the next treatment session; this is like
learning to play the piano — regular practice between lessons being
essential. In cognitive and dynamic therapy also, what he has learnt
intellectually must become his own experience emotionally and able
to be acted upon. It is more straightforward to practise in vivo
control over simple behavioural symptoms; practising appropriate
rather than neurotic patterns of relationships are much more difficult.

Alongside learning self-control is acceptance of how other people function. The neurotic often feels himself to be unique. He needs to realise that the same rules govern his behaviour as others', and that he has the same obligations to other people. It is beneficial for the neurotic for his own treatment to practise thinking about other people and how he can help with their needs.

> 'It's an useful way if you can, to engage them in
> comforting others, that are in deeper Distresses than
> themselves. For this will tell them, that their Case
> is not singular, and they will speak to themselves,
> while they speak to others.'
>
> (Richard Baxter, 1615-1691)

The Problem of Guilt

A person may feel profoundly guilty in a situation where, knowing what is right and what is wrong, he has done what he knows to be wrong. Much more rarely, usually in the context of an endogenous depressive illness and not in neurosis, a patient may have inappropriate delusions of guilt. An 80-year-old man believed that every police car driving along the main road outside his window was looking for him to take him to prison because he had panicked at the front-line, and run away in the 1914–18 war. This conviction had developed over the previous six months; there were other signs of depressive psychosis; his symptoms cleared with treatment.

A person feels guilty because he has done wrong in his own estimation. We do not help him at all by denying guilt based upon his values of right and wrong. We may consider that his conscience (or superego) is overworking, but his feelings can only be dealt with by what he considers to be an appropriate process; treatment involves forgiveness and restitution not denial of guilt. If he can put right what he had done wrong, this is the first step; if not, he should look for a substitute form of restitution. In order to be at one with his community, he needs to believe himself to be forgiven. Some of the most intractable feelings of guilt occur when the victim of the action about which the person feels guilty had died. Restitution and forgiveness from somebody else then becomes necessary: this may be the child of the victim or the social group from which the victim came.

Severe feelings of guilt are very common in neurosis. They need to be accepted as 'real', and dealt with in the context of the patient's own belief and principles; denying a patient's guilt devalues him as a person and undermines his confidence in the therapist.

Options in Treatment

The therapist demonstrates his respect and regard for the patient by providing a comfortable and aesthetically pleasing setting for treatment; that this is beneficial is generally recognised by psychotherapists, who take considerable trouble in planning the 'therapeutic milieu'. An unpleasant, drab or dirty room even though not the fault of the therapist may undermine the relationship with the patient and the latter's ability to achieve self-esteem. 'This is what I have come down to; this is all I am fit for.'

The status of treatment — whether as an in-patient, a day patient or an out-patient — has to be considered. Is treatment active or supportive? Active treatment whether psychodynamic, cognitive or behavioural will be aimed at change. Supportive treatment assumes the patient to have some degree of permanent disability and aims to maximise his potential within these limitations. Treatment that is intended to be supportive by making the best of difficult circumstances may reinforce him in a role of being ill and so retain him in disability.

This needs thinking through; supportive therapy necessarily implies some degree of dependence. Is this the best that can be expected for this patient, or should a more active and perhaps threatening form of treatment be tried?

There is then:

(1) active treatment aimed at improving the patient's condition so that he no longer requires treatment,
(2) supportive therapy that enables him to function through a difficult period of his life and,
(3) there is also treatment that maintains the patient free from symptoms but dependent upon the therapist.

It is important to decide which of these is taking place during treatment.

To understand how relationships work; what is his effect upon other people; and how they, therefore, react towards him, is useful in treatment. He has compensated for his desperate fear of loss of self, by single-minded concentration upon himself and his own concerns. 'Modelling' plays an important part in learning how to relate. To be a suitable 'model', the therapist must be a relatively normal person (not super-human!), exposed to problems, capable of establishing reasonable relationships, and coping with his own life adequately. For most types of treatment, the therapist will need to show his own face, and be a person with distinctive character. The more active is the treatment situation the more opportunity the patient has to witness the therapist's behaviour, and so model his own behaviour and attitudes on the actions of the therapist. An example of this ability of the therapist to show a human face was the occupational therapist who littered her office in the clinic with a jumbled collection of pop-art bric-a-brac. This was not done self-consciously to influence patients; it was simply an expression of her self-confidence as an independent person.

During the process of treatment it is important that the patient has hope for improvement; that he sees this as a real possibility. What is often called lack of motivation may simply be that the patient no longer believes any beneficial change is possible. This hope must be communicated by the therapist, but this can only happen when the therapist is confident in his ability to help the patient.

Preventive Action

Ideally this would be a detailed and lengthy section but lack of firm knowledge about causes and the efficacy of preventive measures makes discussion of prevention highly speculative. Adequate research into the process and outcome and the effects of treatment are essential. Prevention must be concerned with the causes of neurosis. This implies prevention of neurotic reactions by developing methods of dealing with stresses, for instance, in bereavement counselling and also enquiry into aspects of prone personality and how they are influenced by upbringing. It is not possible to remove the causes of stress in society, nor to produce a Utopian society without members who show personality disorder. An important area is the prevention of chronic disability by developing methods and services for early effective treatment.

The responsibility for prevention of neurosis will rest much more with general practitioners than psychiatrists (Royal College of General Practitioners, 1981). Unfortunately there are still many general practitioners who have had minimal training in psychiatry and still quite a few who are not very interested in their neurotic patients. Even when future family doctors have had considerable experience in psychiatry, perhaps six months of a Rotational Training Scheme, the emphasis may have been much more upon the treatment of psychosis in hospital rather than neurosis in the community. It seems probable that the best way of improving the standard of practice would be to imitate the Court Report (1976) which advocated the establishment of a cadre of general practitioner/paediatricians. The time has come when there should be general practitioner/psychiatrists also. These should not be self-styled experts who have carried out some sessions in a mental hospital over many years, but have no other qualifications. They should be specifically pre- pared for this function, and undergo further training for 3 or 4 years after qualification, in general practice and psychiatry together to equip them for such a role.

Improving the State of the Individual within Society

On looking at which features are pathoplastic in society, it is the individual response to particular circumstances which is important. For example, 'precipitating factors' will have different values in different societies, and in different groups within society. There is, in fact, less bereavement in our society than in the past, but people still experience loss provoked for example, by separation and divorce, and by greater social mobility. It is very difficult to compare whole societies to assess which circumstances cause neurosis.

What we do know about communities is that where morale is high, this helps the individual and lower rates for neurosis are usually found; conversely social disorganisation with the breakdown of families, the run down of industry and high levels of unemployment are associated with higher rates. Public attitudes towards relationships are important, for instance, an attitude of society that treats separa- tion and divorce lightly is likely to be associated with increased separation, and consequently more fractured relationships. This does not only promote neurotic reactions in the marital partners but, more importantly in the children of the marriage. Durkheim's description of *anomie* (1897), that is where people live outside the social mores of a close knit society, is found to be associated with highter rates of suicide. There appears to be an association between higher rates for neurosis and urban working class life, and there is a lower rate in closely knit rural communities. There is perhaps an ideal size and type of structure for communities, which demonstrate low neurosis rates, but such a contention is highly speculative.

Most of the emphasis in the prevention of neurosis will be for the individual case rather than society. Measures to promote self- esteem are likely to be prophylactic, as are factors strengthening relationships. Thus marital therapy can be seen as prophylactic, not only for the partners but also for their children. Work problems are important in the development of neurosis. Dissatisfaction at work and the feelings of worthlessness associated with unemploy- ment are provocations for neurosis. An attitude that regards em- ployment, a sense of achievement, and job satisfaction as important, is beneficial.

An attempt to prevent childhood and adolescent anxiety states can be made by attention to the following points (Royal College of General Practitioners, 1981):

(1) Parents should be encouraged to express their grief following miscarriage or stillbirth, and their emotional state assessed during the following pregnancy.
(2) Complication of pregnancy and the mother's concern for the future of the baby should be discussed openly.
(3) Contact between mother and child after delivery should be encouraged.
(4) Over-close mother/child relationships should be identified and ways found of increasing the emotional support given to the mother in other ways.
(5) General practitioners should encourage over-protected children to return to school as soon as possible after minor illness.

Prevention of personality disorder is very difficult but combating adverse social factors is important. Doctors and social workers should be trained to identify homes where there is a lack of warmth and affection in order to provide more professional support and also aim to strengthen links with family and friends.

Another important way of aiming to prevent neurotic reaction is to anticipate distress during 'psychosocial transitions' (such as separation from parents, marital breakdown, loss of a job, retirement, and so on) and seek to help the individual to cope with this. Preparing people for life events that are likely to prove stressful has been beneficial in some situations. The victim needs to know what will actually happen and what his response is likely to be. It takes time to adjust to such information and rehearsing the plans is helpful. The patient should be encouraged to express his feelings when in a secure setting. Reassurance of the patient's capacity to cope is useful.

During a life crisis which could well precipitate neurotic symptoms, skilled support has proved beneficial to those particularly at risk. Support in such a crisis both implies allowing the expression and discussion of emotion, and the emotionally charged events, and allowing the victim dependence upon another person. A general practitioner who had scarcely seen a middle-aged man who was a patient of his found himself seeing this patient about weekly for six months after his wife's death from cancer. Eighteen months after the death, the doctor realised that he had only seen this patient twice in the last year. The final stage of such support is to help the person find a new adjustment to life.

Early effective treatment of a neurotic reaction, which may

mean referral to an appropriate specialist, will sometimes prevent long term suffering and neurotic disability. If psychotropic drugs are prescribed, these should always be accompanied by counselling or psychotherapy from the doctor.

There are quite a few practical steps that may be taken in the prevention of self-poisoning:

(1) Recognition of those at risk, for example, those who are impulsive, socially isolated, in some sort of severe distress, and have previously taken an overdose.

(2) If suspected, a patient should always be asked if he feels suicidal.

(3) The approach of the therapist in counselling or psychotherapy should be to maintain hopefulness (helping the patient to see what areas of success there have been) and avoid rejection. This does not mean that the doctor should be manipulated by his patient but he should allow reasonable access by giving a further appointment.

(4) When drugs are used, the principles should be to avoid high dosage or dangerous drugs, to prescribe in smaller quantities, if in doubt give the prescription to a relative. Drugs should not be left lying around after use, as many overdoses are of tablets prescribed for another relative.

(5) It is useful to be able to provide a telephone number that the patient can ring if he is desperate. The Samaritans provide such a service. In general practice, this is as much a life and death crisis as many other night calls the practitioner on call may receive. As psychiatric hospitals shift their emphasis from the institution to the community, so this type of crisis intervention will increasingly be seen as part of their function.

(6) If there is clear suicidal risk, psychiatric referral should be seriously considered. Methods of treating, or at least helping, with social conflicts will be necessary as parasuicide is characterised by the florid nature of the social disturbance (Kreitman, 1979).

Research and the Effects of Treatment

There is clearly a need for the application of commonsense, uncontaminated by political motivation, in the planning of society's welfare measures. There is a considerable need for further research into factors affecting the development and the outcome of neurosis. This should aim at investigating both individuals and their communities.

The final and most important question for prevention is, does treatment for neurosis work? If it does then the most significant preventative measure is that those affected be adequately treated, and that those prone receive early help. If treatment can be effective then, of course, the onus for providing treatment becomes very heavy for society. Again this calls for research in evaluation of treatment and in assessing what particular parts of treatment, what methods and strategems are effective. Such research is particularly important in evaluating the claims of the various schools of psychotherapy, according to Shepherd (1979) who quotes Foster (1971), 'those who feel they need psychotherapy tend to be the very people who are most easily exploited: the weak, the insecure, the nervous, the lonely, the inadequate and the depressed, whose desperation so often is such that they are willing to do and pay anything for some improvement of their condition . . . the possibilities of harm to the patient from the abuse, or the unskilled use, of these techniques are at least as great as the possibility of good in the right hands'.

Bibliography

Bandura, A. (1978). Modelling. *Adv. Behav. Res. Ther.*, 1, 237–269

Baxter, R. (1691). The signs and causes of melancholy. With directions suited to the case of those who are afflicted with it. Collected out of the works of Mr. Richard Baxter for the sake of those, who are wounded in spirit. By Samuel Clifford, minister of the Gospel, 1716, Cruthenden & Cox, London

Bird, J., Marks, I.M. and Lindley, P. (1979). Nurse therapists in psychiatry, controversies and implications. *Br. J. Psychiat.*, 135, 321–329

Court, S.D.M. (1976). Fit for the Future: Report of the Committee on Child Health Services (Command Papers 6684), H.M.S.O., London

Durkheim, E. (1897). Le Suicide (Trans. 1952: *Suicide: a Study in Sociology*), Routledge & Kegan Paul, London

Foster, J.G. (1971). *Enquiry into the Practice and Effects of Scientology*, H.M.S.O., London

Frank, J.D. (1974). The restoration of morale. *Am. J. Psychiat.*, 131, 271–4

Gelder, M. (1979). Behaviour therapy as self-control. In: *Current Themes in Psychiatry 2* (Ed. Gaind, R.N. and Hudson, B.L.), MacMillan, London

Kreitman, N. (1979). Reflections on the management of parasuicide. *Br. J. Psychiat.*, 135, 275–277

Marks, I.M. (1974). Research in neurosis: a selective review 2 Treatment. *Psychol. Med.*, 4, 89–109

Royal College of General Practitioners (1981). *Prevention of Psychiatric Disorders in General Practice*, Royal College of General Practitioners, London

Seabrook, M.F. (1973). A study of the influence of the cowman's personality and job satisfaction on the milk yield of dairy cows. *J. agric. Lab. Sci.*, 1, 49–93

Shepherd, M. (1979). Psychoanalysis, psychotherapy and Health Services. *Br. med. J.*, 2, 1557–1559

Truax, C.B. and Carkhuff, R.R. (1967). *Toward Effective Counselling & Psychotherapy: Training & Practice*, Aldine, Chicago

11 Methods of Treatment

'Reflecting today on the case of a poor woman who had continual pain in her stomach, I could not but remark the inexcus-
able negligence of most physicians in cases of this nature. They
prescribe drug upon drug without knowing a jot of the matter
concerning the root of the disorder. And without knowing this
they cannot cure, though they can murder, the patient. Whence
came this woman's pain (which she would never have told had
she never been questioned about it)? From fretting for the
death of her son. And what availed medicines while that fretting
continued? Why, then, do not all physicians consider how far
bodily disorders are caused or influenced by the mind?'

John Wesley; Diary, May 12th, 1759

No one general practitioner will have all methods of treatment available to him, even less will he be able to practise them all himself.
Here follows a brief description of some of the myriad treatments. In
figure 11.1 is shown the decisions a doctor might make in choosing
a method of treatment. Of course, different methods are not necessarily exclusive.

Treatment by Psychotherapy

What is psychotherapy? There are many definitions of psychotherapy
and the word may be used in a limited sense according to the practice
of a particular school of treatment, or in a much wider sense referring
to all 'talking treatments'. Psychotherapy includes all structured
methods of improving individual wellbeing by use of human relationships. Clearly, verbal communication is important, but non-verbal
methods may also be used, for instance in gesture, human contact or
in mime and drama. Improving individual wellbeing is an aim in
many relationships; psychotherapy implies skill acquired by special
training undertaken by the therapist. Training will grant official
recognition by a respected organisation; it should allow the possibility
of theoretical explanation of the causes of conflict, and ensure
accepted standards of practice of treatment.

Psychotherapy is practised at different levels. In one sense all
doctors must be psychotherapists, as they need to use their relationship with the patient to help him. Most of a psychiatrist's time in
contact with patients is occupied by psychotherapy; there cannot,

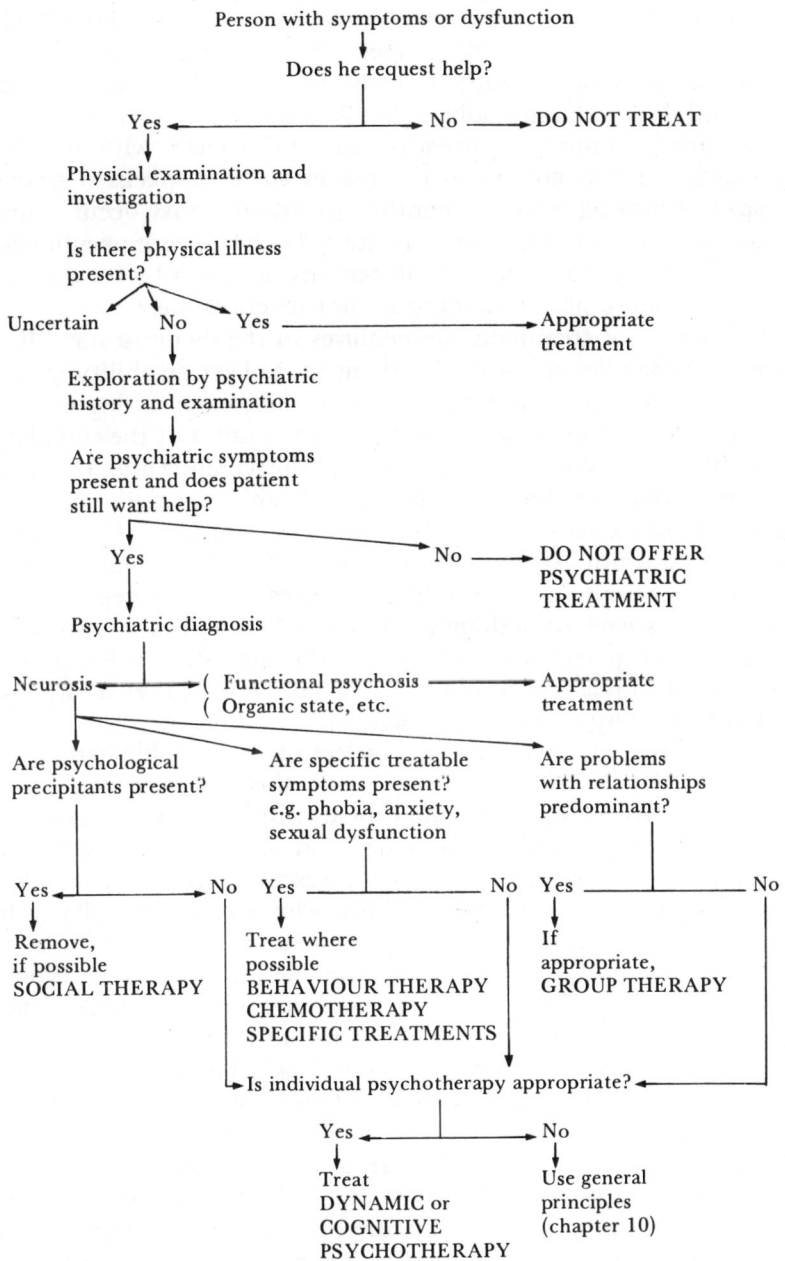

Person with symptoms or dysfunction

Does he request help?

Yes ← | → No → DO NOT TREAT

Physical examination and investigation

Is there physical illness present?

Uncertain — No — Yes ————————→ Appropriate treatment

Exploration by psychiatric history and examination

Are psychiatric symptoms present and does patient still want help?

Yes — No → DO NOT OFFER PSYCHIATRIC TREATMENT

Psychiatric diagnosis

Neurosis ← | → (Functional psychosis ————→ Appropriate
(Organic state, etc.   treatment

Are psychological precipitants present?   Are specific treatable symptoms present? e.g. phobia, anxiety, sexual dysfunction   Are problems with relationships predominant?

Yes — No   Yes — No   Yes — No

Remove, if possible SOCIAL THERAPY   Treat where possible BEHAVIOUR THERAPY CHEMOTHERAPY SPECIFIC TREATMENTS   If appropriate, GROUP THERAPY

Is individual psychotherapy appropriate? ←

Yes — No

Treat DYNAMIC or COGNITIVE PSYCHOTHERAPY   Use general principles (chapter 10)

Figure 11.1   Treatment decisions in neurosis

or should not, be a psychiatrist who is not also a psychotherapist. However, there is also further specialism in a particular mode of psychotherapy which enables a person with such experience to train others and deal with especially difficult situations.

This brief account is intended for the doctor who is not a psychiatrist; it will not equip the reader to be a specialist psychotherapist. Knowing what psychotherapy is, and what occurs during the course of treatment, is no mandate to launch oneself unsupervised into disturbing the equilibrium of patients, however faulty that may be. Many types of psychotherapy are not described here.

In all forms of treatment the qualities of the therapist himself are paramount (Sandler *et al.*, 1973). He needs to have an ability to communicate; this implies listening to the patient, empathising with the distress he is describing, analysing the main features of the complaint, attempting to understand this in terms of the patient's life experience, and verbalising his formulation. Considerable demands are made upon the therapist's own stability of personality. He requires emotional warmth, without potentially harmful over-involvement. For psychotherapy to proceed, it is necessary to accept that all human beings have something in common that allows one to generalise from one person to another. Another necessary assumption is that defined causes will produce predictable effect; that is, stimulus is followed by response in human affairs.

In all types of psychotherapy selection of suitable patients is imperative (Bloch, 1979). Motivation is the first requirement for suitability. Victims of acute situational crisis form the majority of clients for non-medical counselling, and when the crisis resolves improvement becomes likely. The neuroses and long-term personality disorders form the majority of those who receive formal psychotherapy. The YA(R)VIS patient has sometimes been regarded as the ideal for psychotherapy; that is, the patient should be young, attractive (rich) verbal, intelligent and successful. However, more carefully conducted outcome studies have shown that age is relatively unimportant; many therapists achieve satisfactory results with middle aged patients. Many methods of treatment have concentrated upon middle-class patients with verbal fluency; programmes are being devised now to help those who are less verbal. One important dimension that appears to have a bearing upon success and therefore for selection of patients is the feature of 'psychological mindedness'. Those who are able to conceptualise their own problems in psychological and emotional terms, and communicate their dissatisfaction with themselves are more likely to respond to treatment than those who are only able to formulate their distress in terms of somatic symptoms. If psychotherapy is a specific form of treatment for

Table 11.1 Some established forms of psychotherapy

Activity therapies (art, dance, drama, music, etc.)	Implosion therapy
	Marital therapy
Anxiety control training	Meditation
Behavioural modification	Modelling
Biofeedback with therapy	Negative practice with conditioned inhibition
Brief psychotherapy	
Cognitive therapy	Operant conditioning
Conditioned aversion therapy	Play therapy
Crisis intervention	Psychoanalytic therapy
Dynamic psychotherapy	Reciprocal inhibition
Experimental therapy	Relaxation therapy
Existential psychotherapy	Sex therapy
Family therapy	Social rehabilitation
Group therapy	Supportive therapy
Hypnotherapy	Work rehabilitation

neurosis it should work as well in severe neurosis as in mild, but does it?

A conceptual framework for psychotherapy is necessary for communication to proceed. It helps the patient to have confidence in his therapist knowing that understanding his conflict conforms to a general theory; and it retains the intellectual curiosity of the therapist in matching the description he receives from his patient with his theoretical predictions. The therapist plans his treatment partly in conformity with his theoretical stance, but also according to his own views as a person, his philosophical standpoint, world view, and religious (or a-religious) beliefs. Several references have been made to the diversity of psychotherapy. To demonstrate this a few of the reputable types of therapy are listed in table 11.1.

Dynamic Psychotherapy

Psychotherapy in its present form originated in psychoanalysis, some of the bases of which are described with a recommendation that the possible relevance of this theory is borne in mind for the individual case. Dynamic psychotherapy makes the assumption that the patient's problems arise within himself and not solely as the effect of external circumstances operating upon him.

The psychoanalytic school has had a relatively small effect upon British psychiatry, and its adherents treat only a minute proportion of all neurotic patients. This is partly because the majority of patients are treated within the National Health Service where psychoanalysis is almost unobtainable, and partly because of the traditional links between psychiatry, in Britain, with the rest of medicine.

In classical Freudian theory, all present problems are seen to have their origins in early sexual conflict. For example, a boy aged 3 or 4 has sexual thoughts and fantasies concerning his mother, but on acting upon these thoughts (or even thinking pleasantly about them), he feels disapproved by adults, and made to feel guilty. The sexual thoughts and feelings, and also the experience of conflict and feelings of guilt are forcibly removed from consciousness; that is, they are 'repressed'. These repressed ideas have little influence upon him for the years up to puberty, but they may interfere with his establishing heterosexual relationships in early adult life. He may be unable to make a long term close relationship leading to marriage, and may substitute for this furtive promiscuity or homosexuality. All other conflicts, including those that are not overtly sexual are also seen as arising from early sexual conflict. Symptoms are removed by bringing into consciousness the meaning of these events that have been long repressed.

Freud conceptualised the parts of the self in almost physiological terms; *Ego* is similar to *self*, as I see myself; *Superego* is closer to the traditional concept of conscience; and *id* like the idea of instinct. These different parts exist in dynamic equilibrium; but in neurosis are in conflict. So the dominant superego of the obsessional acts as a censor upon his behaviour. Psychopathic behaviour occurs because of insufficient control by other levels upon the activity of id. Conflict, with psychological defences established so that feelings of anxiety are not experienced, is not necessarily pathological, it occurs in normal non-neurotic people as well.

A most important tenet of Freudian theory is the influence of unconscious mind on the whole of a person's experience and behaviour. We have already discussed how repression occurs and contents of consciousness in early childhood become unconscious. Freud saw this removal of material from conscious awareness to the unconscious as being an active process, so that forgetfulness or slips of the tongue were not accidental or meaningless, but were a glimpse into the unconscious mind. Much of the technique of psychoanalysis is aimed at making unconscious material accessible to conscious thought and present day emotion by helping the patient to explore these repressed conflicts using the relationship with the therapist as a defence against the fear thereby engendered.

The patient resists the removal of this censorship unconsciously produced; it is a painful process. Treatment proceeds with confrontation of the unconscious mechanism, clarification and interpretation. Feelings of anxiety are experienced when the emotion from the conflict is felt without the cause of the conflict becoming conscious. A person protects himself from this anxiety by various 'ego-defence mechanisms'. These prevent the experience of anxiety and hence allow the person to function despite the presence of unresolved conflicts. In neurosis the defences partly fail to repress conflict into unconsciousness and symptoms occur as a distorted representation of the inner struggle.

The classical method of exploration of personal conflict in psychoanalysis is by free association. The patient is asked to say everything that comes into his head immediately, without the usual reticence that results from thinking what the consequences would be. This is a technique for revealing material that is unconscious and usually censored.

The therapeutic relationship in psychoanalytic treatment is of vital importance. A female patient may unconsciously transfer positive feelings which she experienced in childhood towards her father, now, in the therapeutic relationship, towards her therapist. She accepts what he says and is concerned to impress him with her enthusiasm to cooperate in treatment. It is not he as a person who is invested with this 'transference relationship', but his role as therapist and, hence, person in authority. In *transference*, the therapist takes on the emotional role of a previous significant person in the life of the patient. The transference element of the relationship should be recognised and used to establish a therapeutic alliance. In time this part of the relationship must be worked through to avoid incapacitating dependence.

Negative transference describes the hostile feelings that the patient may have experienced towards a significant adult being transferred to the therapist. Without his saying a word a young woman comes into the doctor's room, kicks his desk and tells him, 'You just sit there looking smugly at me. You hypocritical stuffed shirt; it's all very well for you'. Negative emotions were transferred unconsciously to the therapist, and the doctor involved subsequently explored her feelings of resentment against her overbearing father. As well as the patient being influenced by previous relationships, the therapist is also, and this is called *counter-transference*. Similarly, negative feelings of the therapist towards his patient because of his previous conflict involving a significant person is called *negative counter-transference*. The transference relationship matters, but it is important to retain proportion; there is also a non-transference relationship, the patient may dislike her doctor because he is rude, arrogant and un-helpful. A triangle of insight has been described (Menninger, 1958), in which the patient's relationships are explored towards the therapist, towards other people of significance in his present life and towards important people in his distant past.

The transference relationship is examined and interpreted in psychoanalytic therapy and the patient comes to see its significance. In exploring defence mechanisms the patient learns about himself and how he can deal with repressed unconscious material. Freudian analysis has concentrated considerably upon the dreams the patient describes during the interview; these are interpreted. Early in his career, Freud experimented with hypnosis as a method of obtaining information from his patients, but later he concentrated upon free association.

Psychoanalysis is extremely demanding in time, and hence expensive. A course of treatment may take place for 50 minute sessions 4-5 times each week, and this may continue for a matter of years. In practice, therefore, it is a useful method of training for psychotherapists, but has little relevance for the majority of sufferers from neurosis. Its importance is partly historical and partly theoretical, with its interest in unconscious motivation and the prominence of sexual conflict.

Psychoanalytic theory has developed in many different directions. We cannot here do more than list a few approaches to treatment:

(1) 'Analytical psychology' based upon the work of Jung; this has been especially concerned with symbolism and the 'collective unconscious';

(2) 'Ego psychology' has resulted from the explorations of Anna Freud into 'ego defence mechanisms'; such as 'projection', 'denial' and 'intellectualisation';

(3) 'Object relations theory' has been concerned with the effect of interpersonal relationships, the development of emotional bonds, and also the effects of loss and attachment as exemplified by the work of Balint (1968), Bowlby (1969), Fairbairn (1952), Winnicott (1958) and Klein (1948);

(4) 'Interpersonal theory' is particularly concerned with the development of relationships at different ages based upon the work of Harry Stack Sullivan (1953);

(5) 'Existential psychoanalysis' is best known from the work of Jean-Paul Sartre (1943);

(6) 'Client centred psychotherapy' was developed by Carl Rogers (1967) and others.

The more elaborate workings of psychotherapy are a matter for experts. However, there are some implications for the ordinary contact between doctor and patient. The fact that there may be underlying conflicts present, of which the patient is not aware, but which influences every day behaviour, is important. It may not be beneficial to force this into the patient's awareness, but it is worth the doctor keeping these unconscious aspects in mind. Similarly the transference relationship has implications for all doctor-patient relationships, and for how the doctor sees himself as a therapeutic instrument. It is useful to understand the mechanisms a person uses to prevent the experience of anxiety. We live in a very different social climate from Vienna at the end of the 19th century, and in no area has this changed more than in our views about sexual behaviour, worries about sex, and sex as a subject for general conversation. This has radically altered the need for repression into unconsciousness of some conflicts concerning sex, and so few people would now accept the universality of sexual conflict as a cause for neurosis.

An important development of dynamic psychotherapy for the treatment of neurotic (and other) patients in general practice has been the work of Balint (1957). He discussed in considerable detail with many illustrative cases how psychotherapeutic principles and object relations theory could be applied in general practice, and how this would affect the doctor himself. The doctor learns about his own relationships with people in authority (the group leader), with his peers, and with his dependents (his patients).

'Supportive psychotherapy' is different from interpretative, insight-giving psychotherapy. The aim is to use the patient's ego defence mechanisms to help him through a difficult situation; these defences are not interpreted as this would expose him to anxiety, but they are allowed to remain. It is important that this treatment should genuinely support the patient in dealing with long term disadvantage, and not reinforce him in the assumption of a sick role.

Casework is the use of the relationship with a professional therapist in helping with a client's psychological and social problems. It is a term generally used in social work, and so the emphasis is upon dealing with social difficulties and involvement with the person's family or environment group.

There has been an enormous development of *counselling* over the last few years. In this a beneficial relationship is fostered, most often, by a carefully trained volunteer to help those with various types of need. Using a trained counsellor in general practice was found to reduce the need some patients had for psychotropic drugs, and also to diminish these patients' needs for medical time (Anderson and Hasler, 1979). For the professional, cooperation and liaison with counsellors is important so that they can use their time and abilities to the greatest possible effect, and obtain professional advice when needed. Training in some basic principles of psychotherapy is a way in which professional workers can help volunteer counsellors.

Individual psychotherapy of a specialist, dynamic type is limited in its application. It is time consuming and hence expensive, and can only be applied to a minority of people. It requires (i) verbal skills from the patient, (ii) an ability to see areas of conflict in psychological terms and to explore feelings, (iii) at least average intelligence, and (iv) flexibility of approach. The severe neurotic, who is totally drained of optimism or motivation by his feelings of inevitability, will not feel able to work towards change. The application of psychotherapy in neurosis tends to be for the middle area of severity rather than either extremes.

Group Psychotherapy

People live in families, work in offices or factories, and often spend their leisure together with others. Neurotics suffer and cause suffering in their relationships, as well as locked within themselves. It is therefore reasonable that treatment should look at both group and individual processes. Group psychotherapy is particularly useful for forms of disorder that are manifested in a group setting. As well as being more economical in scarce therapist resources, the group emphasises that the patient is not unique in his anguish; other people have somewhat similar problems. It also allows a reflection within the group of the sort of dynamics that occur usually within a family; the leader of the group is likely to take on a 'transference' role for the members, and this can be useful to discuss in treatment. As others resolve their difficulties, so the individual patient begins to realise how improvement can occur.

Groups are valuable for patients with social phobias; that is, those who have difficulty with mixing, who would like to relate better to other people, and feel that others dislike them or notice them in an adverse and critical way. People with schizoid or paranoid personalities are less likely to obtain benefit. The paranoid personality is likely to set himself up in the group as a scapegoat, and then understandably to have persecutory feelings when the other members attack him. The feelings generated within the group may simply not reach the person with schizoid personality cocooned by his withdrawal from human contact.

Groups may be large (more than 25), or small (8-10), structured or unstructured, open or closed. Open groups receive new members and discharge those who have completed their treatment, but the group itself continues; typically it might take place in a psychiatric ward. As the composition of the group changes, so does the emotional atmosphere amongst the members. This is similar to the gradual changes in social dynamics that occur in most natural groups apart from the family. In a closed group, all the members start at the first session with their therapist and remain together until treatment has been completed. This allows distinct phases of group treatment to be identified; the striving for group identity and meaning with attempts to gain the attention of the leader; the stage of active work with different members of the group making progress; resolution of problems with a sense of group cohesiveness. The composition of groups is a delicate matter. There are very diverse theories as to what diagnostic mix should be provided, and what roles within the group the different members should be chosen to fill.

Some therapeutic processes occur more easily in groups than for patients in individual treatment. Cohesiveness is encouraged so that members feel concerned and even responsible for each other (Yalom, 1975). They are involved with the progress of the members and look for ways in which they can help other people. They learn to be sensitive to other's feelings and how their own behaviour affects other people. Interpersonal learning is encouraged in which they come to understand the other's motives and apply this to themselves.

Groups may be used in a number of different settings, for example, in prisons and special units for the treatment of those with severe personality disorders. Group therapy and the therapeutic milieu makes a substantial contribution to psychiatric day care. Many psychiatric wards use group therapy as part of their treatment regimen. More intensive interpretative groups may be used as a vehicle for psychotherapy rather than individual psychotherapy. It is important for the role of the staff members of the group to be clear, and it is necessary for patient groups to be followed by staff discussions of what was happening in the group.

Group therapy like other forms of treatment has potential dangers. There are casualties who sustain harm from participation especially amongst those who have very low self-esteem and very high expectations from the group. Casualties are more likely when the leader is aggressive, intrusive and more concerned with individual rather than interpersonal processes (Yalom and Lieberman, 1971). An important function of the skilled leader is to protect vulnerable members of the group from excessive emotional pressures from their peers.

Role Playing and Psychodrama

There are severe limitations in the application of individual psycho-

therapy; it is expensive, time-consuming, and only one relationship —
that between the therapist and patient — is available for exploration.
Group psychothrapy is less labour intensive, but still depends upon
a verbal exchange between the members of the group and the therapist. There is a need for treatment methods that do not rely exclusively on language, and therefore are more appropriate for people
with less verbal skill, perhaps of lower intelligence, and coming from
a cultural background less concerned with words.

In role playing and psychodrama the patient does not only describe the situation of conflict and problems with relationships
in words, but he acts them in a simulated drama. This may take
place in an individual treatment situation, but more often within
a group. It can be used in quite simple form in treatment; for example, the therapist allows discussion within the group to proceed
for a time in order to create a congenial atmosphere and to collect
suitable material for role playing. A situation from the recent life
experience of a group member may become the scenario for the
drama. This patient, with the leader's help, sets the scene and allo-
cates roles to different group members. The drama then proceeds
with the patient describing its course and the leader producing it.
The purpose of the exercise is to explore the possible feelings of
the different characters in the episode in order to work out why
they acted the way they did, and to practise new ways of coping
with the conflicts that occur in real life.

Psychodrama was brought into medical practice by Moreno in the
1920s (Davies, 1976). Events of emotional significance are enacted
in order to resolve conflict and enable creative activity to take place.
Encounter occurs in a 'here and now' situation with a mutual exchange
of thoughts and intense emotions uncensored. The action of the
drama both repeats the activities occurring at the time of the original
conflict (a patient described, 'when they sent me to Coventry in the
pub because Bill hinted I was homosexual'), and also explores
possible ways of dealing with it. There is an emphasis on trying to
capture the significant moment and also allowing the drama to
proceed in a spontaneous and unscripted fashion. Treatment involves catharsis, that is emotional purging, and gaining insight.
Psychodrama has been developed in various ways by different
schools of psychotherapeutic technique, for example, in 'sensitivity
groups'.

Hypnotherapy and Relaxation

Hypnosis, although one of the oldest techniques in the treatment
of neuroses, is poorly understood. It is a state of heightened suggest-

ibility, artificially induced, and physiologically distinct from sleep. The field of consciousness is narrowed to little more than the thera-- pist and his suggestions and various motor and sensory changes can be induced producing muscular relaxation, paralysis or passivity, numbness and paraesthesiae and also increased attention to fantasy and memory; creation of fantasy is an essential element of hypnosis. There appears to be a covert contract between subject and hypnotist that the former will voluntarily act upon the instructions of the latter, provided the latter does not abuse this by asking the subject to do something unacceptable.

Hypnosis is not treatment in itself but is used as an adjunct to other methods of treatment. It may be used in the investigation of conflicts that are not accessible in interview. A young girl had attacks when she would feel dizzy and fall down. No physical cause was found and she could not describe any emotional factors during interview. However under hypnosis she described her sister's nightdress catching fire four years before, and herself looking on, horrified and intensely guilty, but unable to do anything about it.

Hypnosis can also be used to induce relaxation and lessen anxiety. Various somatic symptoms have been treated in this way including hysterical conversion symptoms. A patient with psychogenic urinary retention was taught relaxation under light hypnosis with an elaborate fantasy of being able to micturate in an unstressed situation. The symptom was successfully treated.

Hypnosis may be used as an abreactive technique. Symptoms may follow terror or extreme anger, and under hypnosis it may be suggested that he relive in fantasy this stressful happening. The resultant extreme emotional discharge, for example, of severe anxiety, may produce catharsis or cleansing with relief of symptoms.

Relaxation can be induced using light hypnosis and then the patient may be taught how to use this technique to produce relief from anxiety somatic symptoms for himself (Snaith, 1981). Autogenic training, or learning to relax oneself at times of feeling stressed can be very useful in the treatment of neurotic symptoms (Schultz and Luthe, 1969).

Behavioural and Other Forms of Therapy

Behavioural Modification

There are no firm rules as to which sort of treatment which patient should receive. Individual or group, dynamic or behavioural; the decision rests with the therapist according to which he considers will most benefit his patient and, of course, which are available. Some of these options are shown in table 11.2.

In behavioural treatments the emphasis is upon what the patient does rather than what he thinks. There are two ways in which such treatments have been developed (Gelder, 1979). First, from learning theory principles, methods of management have been devised. Second, long established techniques of commonsense learning have been systematised to produce improved results (Marks, 1979). Behavioural modification has resulted in methods of treatment that are less demanding of time than dynamic psychotherapy, and may be useful in about an eighth of all psychiatric out-patients. For treatment, a precise description of the maladaptive behaviour is required with analysis of its component parts, and a behavioural regime devised to correct this. Practising behaviour therapy is not confined to any one profession; programmes are often devised by a clinical psychologist or psychiatrist, but increasingly behaviour therapy has become an area of expertise for the nurse therapist. As often as possible, treatment should be carried out *in vivo* with the patient and the therapist rehearsing behaviour in the situation where symptoms normally occur, for example, at home in the bathroom or in a busy shopping street.

The two main theoretical bases for behavioural psychotherapy are Pavlovian *classical conditioning*, and *operant conditioning* as developed by Skinner. Classical conditioning assumes that symptoms are learnt as a conditioned reflex associated with specific behaviour, and treatment requires unlearning by allowing the patient to experience the situation without excessive anxiety. In operant conditioning, it is taken that neurotic symptoms have established a pattern by being reinforced or rewarded. Treatment proceeds by

Table 11.2 Treatment options in neurosis

	Symptoms concerning self-attitudes	Problems with relationships and interaction
Dynamic psychotherapy	Individual psychoanalysis	Group dynamic therapy
	Cognitive therapies	Family, marital therapy, etc.
Behavioural psychotherapy	Behavioural analysis and treatment	Social skills treatment Sex therapy

achieving reinforcement from non-neurotic behaviour, for example, the therapist or better still the patient group, congratulates and reassures the phobic patient with acclaim on her successful return from the supermarket. Of course, this is a gross simplification of a complicated method about which numerous learned articles have been written.

In the treatment of a phobia for birds or feathered objects carried out in vivo, *desensitisation* by *reciprocal inhibition* takes place exposing the patient to a hierarchy of stimuli from nondescript furry objects until eventually a live bird is handled. Desensitisation implies removal of the anxiety which has become the conditioned response to the stimulus of exposure to a bird by a behavioural process which obliterates the conditioned response. *Reciprocal inhibition* means preventing or diminishing the response of anxiety in the presence of an anxiety-provoking stimulus; the inhibition of anxiety is learnt as a response in behavioural modification. It assumes that anxiety is central to all neurotic disturbance and that neurotic behaviours are fundamentally learned or conditioned. Analysis of behaviour in this case entails a precise phenomenological description of what about birds and which birds make the person anxious. Treatment through the hierarchy starts with the least anxiety-provoking situation and proceeds to the next stage only when that situation can be experienced without anxiety. Sometimes the phobic object cannot be produced and so techniques involving fantasy are required. This is necessary for a phobia associated with thunder and lightning, or for flying. Various devices involving 'thought stopping' and treatment in fantasy have been developed for a wide range of different conditions. For example, a patient with distressing and incapacitating obsessional ruminations was asked to wear a rubber band on his finger. When the obsession started he had to pull and release the band, giving himself a jolt, and so breaking his pattern of thought.

Implosion or *flooding* treats the patient by sustained exposure to the phobic object until anxiety diminishes. The stimulus (for example, open space) evokes the response of anxiety, and previously has caused the patient to avoid going out of doors; because of her fear of open places, the phobic patient has taken a longer route rather than go home across the main square. With implosion, she is kept in contact with the anxiety producing stimulus (standing in the square with her therapist), until the response of anxiety, fear and panic has subsided. This technique can be used both for phobic states and for obsessional neuroses. Thus, this phobic woman stood in the square with her therapist beside her until she no longer felt anxious. In obsessional neurosis, a technique of *response prevention* was carried out with a ritual handwasher in which he was not allowed to wash his hands for several hours after touching the bottom of his shoe which he considered contaminated. Previously this action of dirtying his hand would be promptly followed by the response of repeated washing during which his anxiety would diminish. With this treatment anxiety will gradually subside although initially it will be quite intense.

Homework is very important in behavioural treatments in order to maintain confrontation with the stimulus causing symptoms. For example, the ritual hand washer would be asked to practise response prevention by touching a contaminated surface several times a day without washing at home in the period between treatment sessions. Using the patient's relatives in therapy and giving homework reduces substantially the amount of the therapist's time required and increases the effectiveness of treatment. The change of behaviour produced in treatment must be internalised by the patient in order for the beneficial effect to be maintained. What the therapist actually says during treatment sessions is important. He should not recommend the patient to avoid the source of anxiety, but to tackle it in the way which has been learned during treatment sessions.

As well as obsessions and phobic states, other disorders have been treated effectively by behavioural psychotherapy. The Masters and Johnson (1970) technique for sexual dysfunction is an application of behavioural methods of treatment. Marital problems have also been diminished along behavioural lines. At follow-up it was found that directive treatment of behavioural type was most efficacious when compared with interpretative or supportive treatment in marital dysfunction (Crowe, 1973). Other behavioural abnormalities have been treated; for example, stammering using breathing exercises, carrying these out in circumstances increasingly likely to exacerbate stammering.

In other conditions behavioural methods have been attempted with variable success. Sexual deviation with exhibitionists has been treated by aversion and self-regulation. Homosexuality, when there has been a request for treatment, has been effectively modified in some subjects. Behavioural methods have been applied to group treatment. 'Social skills' groups counteract the effects of 'learned helplessness' and help to develop the patient's social functioning. This is practical application of operant conditioning in which socially appropriate behaviour is 'reinforced' or rewarded by the explicit approval of other members of the group. Many of the features of group therapy are incorporated, but emphasis is placed on using the relationships within the group situation to practise appropriate methods of communication in everyday life. This may involve role playing in the group, for example, one member with problems with shyness asking another, acting the part of a shopkeeper, for change to make a telephone call. It may also involve work, carried on outside the group, to be reported back to the other group members for their approval. 'Token economy' methods, in which approved behaviour is rewarded by tokens which can later be exchanged for goods or privileges, have been used in the treatment of psychiatric patients, but predominantly for psychotic rather than neurotic patients.

The selection of patients for behavioural psychotherapy is less restrictive than for interpretative dynamic therapy. Clearly motivation is important, and it is usually assessed when the analysis of the maladaptive behaviour takes place. Behaviour therapy attacks symptoms. It must be possible therefore to identify the symptoms and to know which symptom is prominent. One of the limitations of this treatment is that symptoms change, and it is of the essence of neurosis that a whole range of different symptoms occur at different times revealing underlying neurotic ways of solving problems rather than a single abnormal behaviour pattern.

Biofeedback

Alpha rhythm on the electroencephalogram occurs when the subject is awake but relaxed, usually with his eyes closed. This EEG pattern disappears when the subject becomes alert, for example, by opening his eyes. By using a transducer the EEG tracing can be converted into sound and alpha rhythm produces an identifiable tone. Training to relax may use this feedback from the EEG so that the subject learns to enhance alpha rhythm. This can be used as an addition to other methods of self-control such as autogenic training. This whole mechanism of giving the individual information about his biological processes in order, eventually, to control them to his advantage is called biofeedback.

Other biological systems have been used to give the subject information about himself. Tension headaches have been treated by recording from the frontalis muscle of the forehead. Using the transducer to convert electrical activity of muscle into sound, relaxed condition of the muscle produces an occasional bleep, but if the muscle is contracted a rapid emission of sounds occurs. The aim is for the subject to learn how he can relax his frontalis muscle by encouraging behaviour (and state of mind) that produces only occasional bleeps; the patient teaches himself this skill. Blood pressure and skin resistance have been controlled using biofeedback in a similar way. There is scope for the development of such techniques in many physical symptoms occurring in neurotic patients.

Portable units for self-teaching have been used in practice, but more sophisticated polygraphic apparatus is required for research. A physiological function such as muscle tension or skin temperature is constantly monitored; this information is processed or transduced; a continuous feedback of this information, either visually on a screen or as an audible tone, is given to the patient (Kogeorgos and Scott, 1981).

Activity Therapies

Almost every activity that has taken place either accidentally or deliberately in the psychiatric clinic has received the suffix 'therapy'. Thus there is music-, art-, and drama-therapy, various forms of movement, gymnastic and dance therapy and any number of others often taking place within a place, or an allocation of time, known as Occupational Therapy.

These treatments are valuable but it is probable that their value is something they have in common rather than anything specific to the particular activity. Work, and to be occupied, is beneficial. Having nothing to do, boredom and inactivity provokes the neurotic into gloomy introspection and dissatisfying fantasy.

Creativity is an important component in therapy. Art therapy should produce something visually; in music therapy music is made, not just listened to. The activity is enjoyable in itself and the sense of creating something is rewarding. It is also valuable for the person to be totally absorbed in what he is doing.

Part of the value of many of the activities is that they help the patient to relax. The concentration on one specific goal, and ceasing to think about problems and symptoms, allows other parts of the body not involved in activity to be relaxed. There is also a passive side to these occupations, such as, for example, listening to music as an adjuvant to relaxation. From the behavioural standpoint, it is good practice for the person with sleep disorder and fear of insomnia to learn to associate relaxation with something pleasant.

Modelling is an important part of such therapy (Bandura, 1978). The staunchest advocate of music therapy in her very enthusiasm for the subject provides a useful model for patients who, in imitating her, take on some of her attitudes and so benefit from the activity.

These activities are also excellent as goal-directed forms of group activity. They encourage cooperation and thinking for others in the group. They may allow a certain amount of interpretation of others' productions in an unthreatening way which is useful to the person concerned, and so facilitate the work of the group.

Family Therapy

It is very much the emphasis of this book that neurosis both occurs because of pressures in the society outside the individual, and also produces disturbance in this society. The most important social unit is the family. As neurosis is so intimately involved with the well-being of the family it is appropriate that treatment should aim to help the family and not just the individual.

Family therapy works on the premise that a disordered individual will result in a 'sick' family which, in its turn, will precipitate symptoms in individual members of the family. Treatment should therefore be given to the whole family to deal with these disturbed processes rather than solely to the individual with symptoms. Like individuals, families develop through different stages; using this metaphor, courtship is equivalent to the 'conception' of a family, then comes the stage of the partners being on their own, the gradual arrival of children in the family, the maturity of the children, their leaving home, the return to two partners living on their own, and finally dissolution of the family in death of one or other partner. On this basic pattern, family disorder may manifest.

Families may be 'healthy' or 'disturbed' and there are a variety of ways of classifying abnormality. Therapy is aimed at change in attitudes and behaviour within the family group, and will often involve the whole family group in treatment sessions. A careful analysis of the functioning of the family and the contribution of each member to this state must precede intervention. Formulation will delineate the abnormal processes, and also what model of functioning this family uses. The therapist can first work out with all the family a scheme or map of family interactions, then formulate plans to correct the unsatisfactory relationship or systems within the family. This plan is then carried out both during treatment sessions and practised at home. The therapist meets with the family to assess success in achieving changes. Both the family members and the therapist evaluate change in achieving specific goals and general improvement in relationship.

Cognitive Therapy

This method of treatment has been advocated for depression and has been claimed to produce better results than tricyclic antidepressant drugs both in the short term and at one year (Beck *et al.*, 1979). It would appear to be appropriate for treating neurotic depression. The aim of treatment is to modify the depressive thoughts that are always associated with the emotional disturbance — to the extent that thoughts are 'thinking behaviour', it is a form of behavioural modification.

Compared with drug therapy, treatment is time-consuming, requiring about 20 sessions of 50 minutes each at weekly intervals. The patient records between treatment sessions the negative depressive thoughts that occur, the events that led up to these thoughts, and the mood that accompanied them. During treatment sessions these thoughts are examined and how they logically arise from their antecedents is questioned. The patient examines these ideas himself between sessions and is encouraged to set up (dis)provable hypotheses concerning these thoughts about himself. At the same time he is encouraged to find ways of spending his time that give him a feeling of success. These methods of treatment would seem to be worth considerably more exploration of possible efficacy and range of application.

Treatment of Specific Conditions

A great deal has been written about the different conditions that follow, but it is helpful for completeness just to summarise in a few sentences some of the ways in which treatment differs from neuroses in general.

Alcoholism

At the stage of addictive behaviour with social problems resulting, alcoholism is often a treatable condition (Royal College of Psychiatrists, 1979); it is a sterile argument to discuss whether alcoholism is a disease or not. The first stage in treatment is diagnosis which is based upon the presence of either evidence of physical dependence upon alcohol (withdrawal symptoms such as tremor, fits, or delirium tremens), or social problems directly attributable to the abuse of alcohol. For the diagnosis of alcoholism, the doctor must maintain suspicion of the possibility because the patient is unlikely to volunteer the information. When the doctor is convinced that there is a drinking problem, it is best to confront the patient with his opinion and the supporting evidence. A clear statement of the problem and advice to stop drinking given at a critical time by a physician or a general practitioner may be very effective in helping the patient stop. Obviously motivation is all important and the patient must be convinced of the need to relinquish his habit.

A waiting policy is often useful in the treatment of alcoholism. If the patient does not accept that he is alcoholic, or accepts the problem but believes that he can overcome it without help, it is better to tell him that help is available if he wants, and invite him to come again rather than get involved in a lengthy debate trying to convince him. Treatment can only start when the patient accepts that he has a problem with alcohol, realises that something needs to be done about this, and feels that he cannot correct it himself.

Treatment of alcoholism is in two stages; the acute treatment of alcohol addiction, and helping the patient learn to conduct his life without recourse to alcohol. The physical treatment of withdrawal symptoms will require tranquillising drugs (for example, chlormethiazole), and sometimes vitamin supplements, and the correction of calorie depletion and electrolyte disturbance. The psychological treatment of emotional dependence requires working through the need for alcohol and helping the patient find alternative methods of dealing with conflict. Group treatment is often beneficial in this context and various behavioural approaches have been used. Details of this treatment are a matter for the expert.

In the past total and permanent abstinence was regarded as the only cure for alcoholism. Many alcoholics however wish to be able to drink alcohol within moderation. When previously treated alcoholic patients have been followed up a small proportion have been found who have returned to drinking socially and yet are functioning satisfactorily. Attempts have been made therefore to treat certain selected patients with a drinking problem by the behavioural technique of *controlled drinking*. In this, the patient is taught to recognise the experience he gets with a safe level of blood alcohol and, using operant conditioning, he learns to regulate his drinking not to exceed this.

Anorexia Nervosa

This condition usually occurs in young females, who are 15 times more likely to be affected than males. There is profound loss of weight due to self-starvation and amenorrhorea, which may precede the weight loss. There is a disturbance of feeding with abnormal attitudes towards food, and usually disturbance of self-image, abnormality of gender role, and a fear of losing control of behaviour, especially a fear of being unable to stop eating.

Treatment should be considered in two quite distinct phases. The first is the phase of weight gain which may be a life-saving procedure in, for example, girls of normal height weighing less than 30 kg. The attitude towards the patient initially, then, is one of

treating a purely medical condition — dangerous loss of weight —
without, as far as the patient is concerned, attention to its cause.
In the severe case, admission to hospital, complete bedrest and very
careful observation especially during meals is required. Such patients
are adept at disposing of food through an open window, or down
the toilet or on another patient's tray, or even fixing it with ad-
hesive to the underside of the bed. Phenothiazine tranquillisers
such as chlorpromazine may be useful both for calming an over-
active patient and aiding weight gain; antidepressant drugs are
indicated for those patients with depressive symptoms. The patient
is weighed daily, but it is best for the patient not to be told her
weight. Meals should be high in calories and should be compulsory,
even if it takes hours to eat them. Gradual relaxation of this regime
occurs as weight is gained. This is not presented to the patient as
behavioural treatment — rewards for good conduct — but as medical
management — a dangerously ill patient requiring vigorous treatment,
and as she gradually improves so treatment becomes less intensive.

After the initial weight gain comes the extremely difficult phase
of encouraging the patient to maintain a reasonable weight. This
will be a compromise between her ideal weight based on age and
height, and her desired weight. At this stage psychotherapy is
valuable, and this may be dynamic and interpretative, cognitive
or behavioural in form. In practice, a combination of all these
is often helpful. Relations with other members of the family need
to be explored, especially with the mother, and also family attitudes
towards food; family therapy is often indicated. Behavioural treatment usually takes the form of operant conditioning with the use
of reinforcements for achieving targets. However, anorexic patients
are notoriously devious, and the simplistic use of such reinforcements
as going home for the weekend may be counter-productive, for
example, for the patient who does not get on well with her family
and prefers to stay in hospital.

Marital Dysfunction

In all married neurotic patients, attention will need to be paid to
the marital relationship as the neurotic pattern has its effect here
more than in any other part of life. It is always important to interview the spouse of the neurotic patient: (1) to corroborate the
patient's story, (2) to explore the different emphases that the spouse
stresses, (3) to ascertain how the spouse evaluates the personality
of the patient, (4) to form an impression of the personality and
competence of the spouse, (5) to find out if the spouse loves the
patient; does he/she, in fact, want the marriage to succeed?, (6) to

find out how the patient and spouse deal with the symptoms of the patient and conflicts in the marriage, (7) to determine what the expectations of the spouse are for improvement.

When the patient and spouse have both been assessed it has to be decided what form treatment should take. It may be appropriate for the therapist to see husband and wife together, or an additional therapist who also sees the spouse in individual interviews may be preferable. In this conjoint interview, both partners in the marriage may feel freer to talk, and less threatened by a supposed alliance between the therapist and the other partner. Such interviews can be constructive when both partners have at least some intention of making the marriage work. If one partner is bent upon ending the marriage, joint interviews are likely to be either silent occasions in which confidences are not exchanged, or slanging matches.

Frequently management of marital dysfunction in neurosis will mean helping the patient deal with a broken marriage and its consequences. This may also require work with the patient in coping with the long-standing problem in maintaining relationships that contributed to breakdown. Individual and group methods of treatment are appropriate in different circumstances. The three stages of management in marital dysfunction are: basic counselling to the two partners, more elaborate exploration of the dynamics involved, and sexual counselling. Effective treatment of neurosis is an important aspect of improving the quality of marriage in some instances (Dominian, 1968).

Sexual Dysfunction

There is obviously a great deal of overlap between marital and sexual dysfunction; the marital relationship must be assessed before treating sexual difficulties. Sexual problems may be a consequence of neurosis, and they may also precipitate other neurotic difficulties in relationships.

Treatment of sexual dysfunction begins with the precise analysis of the sexual difficulty — in which partner, or both, what actually happens or fails to happen? Then an examination is carried out looking for other non-neurotic causes of dysfunction, for example, physical causes with diabetes or as a side-effect of hypotensive drugs, psychiatric causes such as depressive illness. Only when these have been excluded does specific treatment of dysfunction proceed.

Sexual behaviour is learned; it is therefore appropriate that behavioural methods based on learning should be used in treatment of dysfunction (Gillan, 1978). Treatment often concentrates on anxiety reduction by desensitisation, the principle of 'giving to get', and learning about sexual experience and practice.

Fear of being unable to function sexually and reach orgasm is a substantial cause of situational anxiety. Previous experience of failure will provoke such fear so that the sufferer may come to associate sexual arousal with severe anxiety, and this anxiety prevents orgasm from occurring successfully. Anxiety reduction involves the teaching of muscular relaxation at each stage through a hierarchy of items which have caused anxiety before intercourse so that the couple do not proceed to the next stage until there is no anxiety at that stage, for example, being naked with the other partner. The aim is to proceed to orgasm without anxiety and resultant muscular tension. Masters and Johnson (1970) have developed techniques in which the aim is to give the other partner sexual pleasure in a relaxed state without the anxiety that has become associated with attempting intercourse. Initially therefore intercourse is prohibited. The technique begins with 'sensate focusing' in which the couple touch and massage each other in non-sexual areas of their bodies. 'Genital sensate focusing' follows in which mutual touching of genitalia occurs without orgasm. A further stage is the experimentation with different sexual positions. Intercourse is not attempted until all the preliminaries have been achieved without anxiety.

Sexual education is often an important part of treatment. Learning about their partner's and their own bodies, and sources of pleasure is important, as also is the use of fantasy in producing arousal. An attitude of mind in which experimentation is accepted is a valuable preliminary to subsequent successful intercourse.

Neurosis in the Elderly

This has been discussed in chapter 9. The chief difference between the treatment of neurosis in old age and in younger patients is the overwhelming importance in the former of physical and social factors. Physical illness is usual in patients with late onset neurosis and amelioration of physical symptoms is an essential — dismissing such symptoms as 'just neurotic' is quite unhelpful.

Recent experience of bereavement, lack of contact with family, and social isolation is common in the elderly neurotic. Treatment requires modifying all possible ways of counteracting this loneliness with visits as appropriate from the doctor, health visitor, home help, district nurse and social worker, and also contact with other organisations such as visiting by members of a church when appropriate. Arranging for the old person to visit a social group outside his home is helpful but it will probably take considerable time and persuasion from the person who is concerned with him to achieve this.

Social Forms of Therapy

Manipulation and Change

Social manipulation has unpleasant overtones of mechanistic abuse of power. However, I use it here deliberately because the patient himself, those with whom he lives, and the organisation or individual who pays for this treatment will all be agreed that treatment has failed, if on completion, his ability to cope with circumstances has not improved. That is not to devalue understanding, but simply to point out that insight is a step on the way to the ultimate objective of change. In social manipulation the patient improves his own social circumstances with active help from the therapist. Although social workers are most frequently involved in this process, it is not restricted to them. Nurses and doctors, provided they have equipped themselves with the necessary information about the patient's social background, can be effective catalysts in social change. The idea of social manipulation includes an enormous range of different acts, from the doctor who helps his patient to get a job as a hospital gardener, to elaborate social skills training with the ultimate object of a significant shift of the patient's role within his family. Not only social workers with a mental health emphasis, but also probation officers and others who are called upon to deal with neurosis in different guises will be involved with such objectives. It would seem that social workers have a special usefulness in helping people with chronic neurosis and that most of their effective time should be spent in practical activities rather than casework (Shepherd *et al.*, 1979).

Five characteristics are important in the capacity of the social worker or other professional to promote social change:

(1) Training is important to learn how social groups interact and how to help the neurotic person gain control of his environment.
(2) The orientation of the professional vitally affects his management. Does he see himself as a guru, passively receiving the confidences of his patient, and reflecting them back altered in words but with no additional resources for coping? Does he see himself as an omnipotent puppet-master pulling strings to get his supplicant-client a job (or even a wife)?, or does he see himself as being alongside the patient involved in the struggle, helping where possible but at the same time ensuring that the patient retains responsibility for his course of actions?

(3) The personal skills of the therapist in communication are important, both in how he relates to the patient, and also to the other agencies with whom he may be involved in social intervention.

(4) Although the over-powering therapist may be harmful in producing excessive dependence from the client, there is a need to have the ability to control social situations. This is what the patient so often cannot do; and if the professional can control the situation initially, he may then hand over responsibility for further action to the patient.

(5) Finally, effective social intervention requires a detailed working knowledge of local conditions. This involves knowing one's way around the mundane and tedious intricacies of the social welfare services. What are the patient's rights and what is available locally?

To be able to improve the patient's freedom of action, the therapist himself must not be too restricted by neurotic traits and motivations. The therapist, whose own neurotic needs require the infantile dependence of the patient upon him or her, may initially give the patient a feeling of support and encouragement, but in the long term will hamper further development.

There is a real dilemma in social intervention. How does the therapist, for example, a social worker, know what is best for a patient? Has the latter become a victim of this social worker's own personal ideology? The selectors of professional helpers have a considerable responsibility in what they should look for, and how they assess whether the required characteristics are present.

Treatment Milieu

Which environment is most likely to benefit this individual patient? Should treatment be as an in-patient or day-patient, or should he attend hospital as an out-patient, see his general practitioner regularly, or go to a totally non-medical setting for help? In answering these questions one should not only be concerned with relief of symptoms, but also with which environment is likely to help most with his social difficulties and problems with relationships. An important factor in assessing the treatment milieu is to consider how the patient's family can be incorporated in treatment. In order for the progress achieved in treatment to be internalised, the patient needs to work out how to apply his changed attitudes and behaviour at home.

The atmosphere of a hospital ward is different from the 'real world', and this makes it difficult for the patient to apply the principles he has learnt, for example, in group therapy, to problems at work. To counteract this an attempt should be made to replicate real life situations, for instance, with role playing or by helping the patient to see how the dynamics within the treatment milieu are in fact 'real'. It is often the social aspects of treatment that neurotic patients have found beneficial. I asked 120 neurotic patients at long term follow-up what part of treatment had helped them most. Amongst the replies were such statements as, 'sitting at meals at a small table with both men and women eating', or 'having to talk to people one has nothing in common with'. These situations had not occurred in the circumstances of life before treatment, but became possible with the special conditions of treatment.

Psychiatric Nursing

I hope that one of the clearest points to come from this discussion of treatment of the neuroses, is the complementary role the different professions have in treatment. No one profession has the monopoly, either in the right to treat or in methods of treatment. Within the psychiatric hospital and increasingly also in the community the psychiatric nurse has a fundamental role. The nurse is often the executive who actually carries out the treatment plan. There has been a radical change of emphasis in psychiatric nursing over the last few years from a custodial to a therapeutic role. Twenty years ago psychiatric nurses very rarely came into contact with neurotic patients, who represented less than 2% of the psychiatric hospital population.

This changing emphasis towards the treatment of neuroses has created a challenge within the psychiatric establishment, as until recently there was little training for nurses in the methods of treatment for neurosis. With improved training, nurses may take on the role of nurse/therapist both in behavioural and dynamic psychotherapy. As for other professions, it is important for the nurse to use herself (or himself) as a person in treating patients. The traditional emphasis in general nursing was to underplay the individual's own characteristics in favour of conformity. Future training of psychiatric nurses will require more emphasis upon therapy both in technique and on the personal demands upon the therapist.

Another recent development is the move for nurses to leave the confines of the hospital for the world outside the walls. They are following the patients, as over the last two decades there has been a dramatic change from long term in-patient psychiatric care towards acute in-patient treatment, with out-patient follow-up and short term readmission as necessary. Community Psychiatric Nursing has developed as a branch of the profession and has a small place in treating chronic neurotic patients.

Treatment from Outside Health and Social Services

Neurosis often presents with physical symptoms or social problems
and it is easy for health or social work professionals to feel that they
carry entire responsibility for coping with neuroses. This is quite mis-
taken as other organisations and institutions help a high proportion
of neurotic people. Traditionally people in Britain looking for help
went to the Church, and nowadays these are not so much the economically poor but 'the poor in spirit' — very often neurotic. Although
this section considers the role of the Christian Church in helping
neurotic people, most of the discussion is equally relevant for other
religions, where the religious organisation forms an important part of
the individual's social life, the minister of religion is a significant
figure, and religious belief influences the individual's attitudes and
behaviour.

Fordham (1953), writing about the work of Jung, commented,
'Many a neurosis can be cured if the sufferer can find his way back
to the Church where he belonged, or experienced a conversion; but
these solutions cannot be imposed, they must arise from the inner
need of that particular person and his awareness and understanding
of that need'. Generally health professionals and religious organisations have had too little to do with each other. They tend to ignore
each other even though they try to help the same people and they
have resources which would be of mutual benefit. Sometimes the
two groups think that their aims and roles are identical; that is that
the Church's goal is to treat symptoms. This is a mistake as most of
the minister's training is not directed towards preparing him to treat
symptoms, and it also implies a surrendering of his vocation as a
minister concerned with spiritual problems.

Religious denominations cannot be emotionally or philosophically
neutral towards psychiatry, nor are psychiatrists neutral in their
attitudes towards the Church. Increasingly ministers are learning in
their training about social organisations such as hospitals, and the application of psychiatry, but unfortunately, psychiatrists remain very
ignorant for the most part about working and functions of the
Church, and the influence belief and also the social structure of the
Church have upon their patients. It is a blind spot in the knowledge
of psychiatrists which probably has its historical origins in the bitter
opposition of the two disciplines in the past.

Because of their feelings of need and their rejection by others,
neurotics are often concentrated in the active community of religious
groups. It is not that the Church makes them neurotic, it is simply
that it is the job of the Church to provide help for those who are
seeking it. Ministers and other workers in religious organisations

therefore need information and training in dealing with neurotic people and this should come from health and social professionals.

It is recognised that some neurotic people get very great assistance in dealing with their problems from their religious beliefs and from the society of the Church. Some are supported so that their long term neurotic disorder causes them less suffering, others are helped to lose their symptoms altogether. The reason why there is a need both for psychiatry and for the Church is that the help that comes from faith cannot be prescribed to order and it cannot be predicted which person with a neurotic disorder will make major progress in the ability to cope following spiritual help.

As well as the value of faith, the neurotic receives benefit from belonging to the Church as a helping, caring, cohesive institution. The strong sense of identity and unity of purpose engendered is of great value. There are many neurotics who are maintained long term and whose further social deterioration is prevented by Church membership. One of the subjects of the study, referred to in chapter 5, of those who were previously treated in hospital for neurosis and were followed up 12 years later, was found to be living in one room in poverty in a deteriorated area of a big city. He was unemployed and extremely isolated, but he spoke of his friends who took him out in their car and invited him for meals. These people proved to be members of the local Roman Catholic Church to which he went; this was almost his only link with other human beings.

A neurotic member of a Church may be helped as follows: First, the minister will have this person forced upon his attention by importunate requests for help, or through difficulties in relationships occurring with other members of the congregation. It is important to decide whether or not there is an underlying neurotic problem, and this may be beyond the minister's competence; in which case professional advice is required. The next stage is to convey to the subject that present behaviour and attitudes are acceptable neither to the person himself nor to others, and that change is possible. There should then be mutual agreement and limited goals for change, for example, coming to Church without disrupting proceedings with histrionic outbursts. The next stage is to support the person as he or she achieves these limited goals using social relationships, and the capacity for mutual caring within the Church. When even limited success is attained this is pointed out to the subject as being the beginning of a process. 'If *this* has been achieved so far, *that* can now be aimed at using the same method.' Ministers are not, and should not aim to be psychiatrists; on the other hand some insight into the mechanisms of neurosis, and also into their own unconscious mechanisms in relationships, is valuable, and an emphasis upon these forms a part of

pastoral training. Psychiatrists can be effective in community psychiatry by maintaining mutually helpful contacts with ministers,
priests, rabbis and other community and religious leaders.

Some of the above principles of management also apply to a lesser
extent to other organisations and societies. This section has taken the
Church as a particular example of how neurosis may be treated outside Health and Social Services. All social organisations with a caring
emphasis tend to attract neurotics amongst their membership, and
these neurotic people both influence the functioning of the organisation and require help.

The Contract for Social Management

Particularly in the social forms of treatment it is important for the
therapist and the patient to agree from the beginning what are the
expectations of treatment. A patient may have quite unrealistic expectations and may have no idea what the therapist can actually do;
the therapist may not know what the patient really wants, and so a
discussion of aims before treatment is essential. Without a clearly
defined agreement, it is very easy for treatment simply to reinforce
the patient in an unsatisfactory social state, with symptoms somewhat diminished or muffled in dependency, rather than achieving
any actual improvement.

Chemotherapy and Physical Methods of Treatment

Like other aspects of treatment for neurosis, drug treatment is an
ideological battle-field (Edwards, 1979). It is very difficult to hold a
balanced and moderate opinion. At one extreme are those who say
that drugs should never be used; at the other are doctors prescribing
purely symptomatically for psychological distress; for example, 18%
of a random community survey in New York were taking sleeping
pills regularly. There is a great need for the use of drugs in neurosis
to be rational. It is a mistake to think that chemotherapy and
psychotherapy are necessarily opposed. Chemotherapy can sometimes be an adjuvant to psychological treatment; the prescription of
drugs should always take into account psychological principles. A
single girl, aged 30 was acting as bridesmaid at her younger sister's
wedding in a few weeks time. She was both fond and envious of her
sister. She complained that she could not sleep. Her doctor understood her conflict over the wedding and discussed this with her; he
also prescribed an hypnotic for 14 days.

Care needs to be taken in the decision whether to prescribe. It is possible that sedating a person may dull the mental discomfort at the expense of preventing him solve his psychological problem by using his own resources (Trethowan, 1975). This may prevent him from coping adequately and so prolong the neurotic disability.

Function of Drug Treatment in Neurosis

Drugs are used in neurosis for the treatment of symptoms. Clearly they can never deal adequately with the difficulties in relationships, with the disturbance of self-image, with the perception of circumstances as stressful nor with abnormalities of personality. Such neurotic symptoms as anxiety, insomnia, depression of mood and psychogenic somatic symptoms are sometimes treated pharmacologically.

Sometimes patients are too disturbed by anxiety to be able to be involved in any type of psychological procedure, and so chemotherapy may precede psychological treatment. Similarly, depression may inhibit concentration, and the subject may be too inert to take part in any behavioural procedure. The prescribing of a drug emphasises the link between doctor and patient, and this relationship once established may then allow psychotherapeutic intervention. There are also problems in this area in that the prescription of a drug may encourage passivity in the patient and raise his expectations that the doctor will 'make him better' without his need for active involvement.

Because of the current expectations of patients, doctors have to make a conscious decision not to use drugs, and so the question is not so much on what occasion drugs should be used, as when they should be omitted. It is important to explain to the patient why he is not receiving medication; why a chemical panacea is not appropriate in non-organic conditions. If no drugs are prescribed it is easier for the patient to accept the explanation that improvement depends upon his altering his behaviour and that improvement is within his own volition.

The use of drugs for different neurotic conditions is not specific. In figure 11.2 are shown the spectrum of use of four of the main groups of drugs: the benzodiazepines, phenothiazines, mono-amine oxidase inhibitors and tricyclic antidepressants. There are a number of newer antidepressants which are not tricyclic in configuration but have approximately the same clinical application.

Action of Minor Tranquillisers and Hypnotics

The benzodiazepine group of drugs are currently the most widely

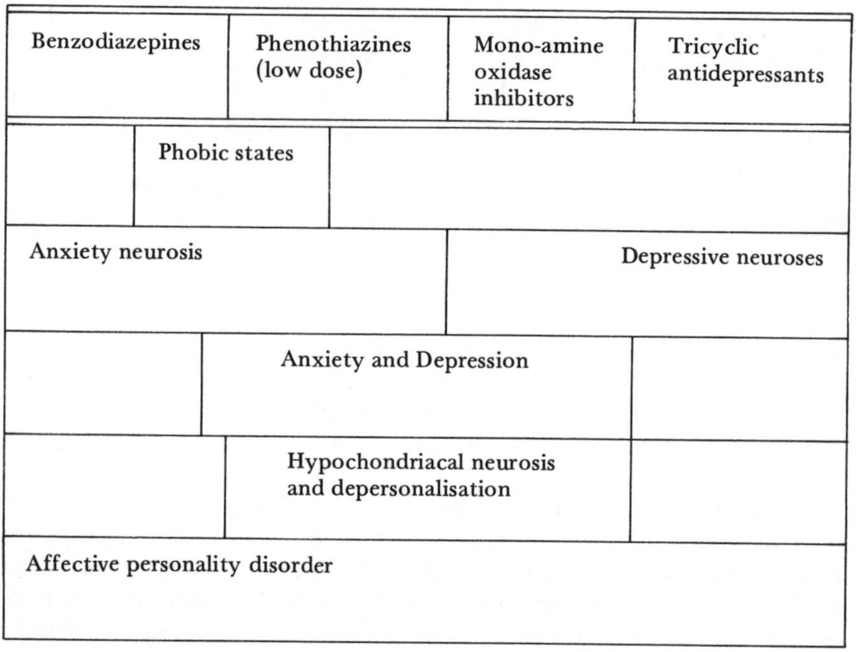

Benzodiazepines	Phenothiazines (low dose)	Mono-amine oxidase inhibitors	Tricyclic antidepressants
	Phobic states		
Anxiety neurosis			Depressive neuroses
	Anxiety and Depression		
	Hypochondriacal neurosis and depersonalisation		
Affective personality disorder			

Figure 11.2   Range of use of drugs in neurosis

prescribed, as centrally acting anxiolytics and also hypnotics; these two uses probably arise from the same pharmacological action — sedation, or inhibition of the Central Nervous System. By 1970, over 15% of the general population were found to be taking them as hypnotics or sedatives in one study. It is probable that sedative hypnotics become ineffective when used nightly in patients over long periods; however, their abrupt cessation will cause withdrawal insomnia (Committee on the Review of Medicines, 1980). Similarly benzodiazepines become ineffective as anxiolytics after more than 4 months use. They have the great advantage of being extremely safe even in vast overdose, and their enormous use has resulted in no direct toxic fatalities and few instances of serious side effects. One danger is their interaction with alcohol to impair performance, for example, driving. Perhaps their greatest disadvantage is the dependence that can become established upon them, and this is more likely for neurotic patients. True addiction is rare but some transitory withdrawal symptoms are described not infrequently. Occasionally they have a paradoxical effect, provoking irritability and aggression instead of tranquillity, especially when there are provoking circumstances. They have been used in neurotic depression but several authors do not consider them superior to placebo in this condition. Benzodiazepines have been effective in the treatment of withdrawal symptoms of alcohol. They are undoubtedly highly effective drugs for the treatment of acute anxiety and sleep disturbance but day-time sedation is often a problem especially with the longer acting drugs which include both diazepam and chlordiazepoxide.

Occasionally major tranquillisers such as haloperidol and chlorpromazine have been used in small dosage for the control of anxiety and other neurotic symptoms. However, even in lower dosage these drugs produce more side effects than the benzodiazepines, and the possible consequences of overdose are much more serious.

More recently Beta-adrenergic-blocking drugs, for example, propranolol, have been extensively used in controlling the peripheral somatic manifestations of anxiety. In the low dosage in which they are used, they have negligible effects upon the central nervous system, but control peripheral anxiety.

Barbiturates were extensively used for the treatment of anxiety but have now largely been superseded because of the very considerable danger, especially in neurotic patients, of habituation and physical dependence. Barbiturates were also a major cause of death through overdosage. Minor tranquillisers, especially the benzodiazepine group of drugs, are quite often useful for the alleviation of acute symptoms in neuroses. However they should never be administered with indefinite 'repeat prescriptions'.

Antidepressants

Are antidepressants drugs effective in the treatment of neurotic depression? Despite a very large number of clinical trials carried out with depressive neuroses there is no clear answer to this question; some studies have found them to be more effective than placebo and others have not. A number of investigators do not make any distinction between neurotic and endogenous depression, but hospital studies include predominantly patients with endogenous depression. Treatment trials carried out in general practice are mostly of neurotic depression; unfortunately the quality of trial has not always been high, and results are variable; we still have no irrefutable evidence for the efficacy of antidepressants with neurotic depression. The dilemma in clinical practice is, on the one hand the gross over-treatment of patients who will never respond to drugs because their symptoms are environmentally caused, and on the other hand the heinous practice of failing to treat a suicidal patient.

Should one use antidepressants in neurosis? If a patient is considered to be suffering from depressive neurosis, it is probably wise to treat with antidepressant drugs under the following conditions:

(1) the patient appears to be quite severely depressed, (2) he fails to improve with measures taken to relieve social difficulties, (3) the condition persists for several weeks, and (4) there is a risk of suicide. It takes at least two weeks for tricyclic antidepressant drugs to begin to have therapeutic effect, and therefore initiating the use of these drugs entails a commitment to continue for at least a month before abandoning as ineffective. Antidepressants should not be seen as a substitute for treatment of the individual using the relationship with the therapist.

Tricyclic antidepressants are those most widely used. They have a proven efficacy in severe depressive illness, but they also have many side effects which means that often patients do not take them in the dose prescribed (see table 11.3). Obsessional and phobic symptoms

Table 11.3 Common side effects with psychotropic drugs

	Symptom	MAOIs	Tricyclics	Benzodiazepine
Interaction with some other drugs with some foodstuffs	Headache and severe hypertensive crisis	+		
with alcohol	Potentiates effects	+	+	+
Endocrine System	Weight gain		+	
Central Nervous System	Convulsions		+	
	Sedation Dizziness		+	+
Autonomic Nervous System	Dry mouth, urinary retention, excessive perspiration		+	
	Blurred vision		+	+
Circulatory System	Postural hypotension	+	+	
	Electrocardiographic abnormalities		+	
Gastrointestinal System	Constipation		+	
Skin	Rash	+	+	+

have been treated with tricyclic drugs; particularly recommended has beem clomipramine. It is likely that these symptoms respond best to tricyclic drugs when there is depression as well as the underlying phobic state.

Monoamine oxidase inhibitors (MAOIs) have also been used in neuroses and they have been recommended for neurotic depression, for phobic states and occasionally in obsessive-compulsive neurosis and hypochondriacal neurosis. Tyrer (1976) considers that patients suitable for treatment with MAOIs cannot be classified using conventional diagnostic labels but include those with primary symptoms of hypochondriasis, agoraphobia and social phobias, irritability, somatic anxiety and anergia. Phenelzine has been found to reduce anxiety but not to affect the phobic symptoms in phobic neurosis. The usefulness of monoamine oxidase inhibitors has been limited because of the severe nature of side effects. When patients taking MAOI drugs eat foods such as some cheeses containing large amounts of tyramine or receive other drugs which are chemically pressor amines, metabolism in the gut by mono-amine oxidase is prevented and these amines are released in the circulation causing hypertensive crisis.

Electro-convulsive Therapy and Psychosurgery

Electro-convulsive therapy is not indicated in the neuroses. However, sometimes a patient suffering from resistant depression which has not responded to other methods of treatment including antidepressant drugs in appropriate dosage has benefited from electro-convulsive therapy. Diagnostic criteria are not sufficiently precise to allow one to be completely certain that a patient will not respond to electroplexy.

The indications nowadays for carrying out psychosurgery for neurosis are extremely rare. It will just occasionally be worthwhile in the very severe chronic neurotic patient. The chief indications are resistant states of tension with obsessionality or depression. Normally the patient will not have been referred for surgery unless there has been sustained disability over several years with failure to gain relief from all other methods of treatment used over an extended period.

A Treatment Plan for the Neurotic Patient

This discussion of treatment has necessarily been discursive and far from complete. Within the space available it has only been possible to give a very brief outline. The following is an abbreviated plan for the treatment of a neurotic patient who might have presented in general practice:

(1) Diagnosis: Is the patient suffering from neurosis? This should be ascertained by the exclusion of physical illness, by the exclusion of other psychiatric conditions: psychosis, organic states or mental handicap, and by the finding of positive features of neurosis. Bearing neurosis in mind as a possibility is a prerequisite for its diagnosis.

(2) Once the diagnosis is reasonably certain avoid further physical investigation and treatment. If the doctor considers the condition to be neurotic but treats the symptoms as physical, this reinforces the position of the patient in the sick role and this may prove a hindrance to treatment.

(3) Assessment of factors relevant for prognosis and treatment is required. For how long has there been neurotic disability? What is the duration of this episode? What are its precipitants? What are the patient's perceived stresses? There should also be assessment of the patient's personality and his social symptoms. Information should be obtained about his social environment at home and at work, and, if possible, another informant interviewed.

(4) The general practitioner, social worker, or psychiatrist should next ask the question: 'Can I achieve the best possible result or should I refer the patient elsewhere?' There is an advantage in working with an already established relationship, but someone else may have greater expertise for this particular sort of problem. Referral should be made for the benefit of the patient not for relief of the therapist. If referred, to whom should it be? This depends both on the type of treatment required and the expected match in personality of patient and new therapist.

(5) The therapist should be clear in his own mind what are the goals of treatment. This depends upon an accurate assessment of the patient's problem and his environment and knowledge of what treatment options there are. Obviously goals set, in terms of achieving understanding and change of behaviour, must be realistic.

(6) The aims of treatment are agreed with the patient. This will be a compromise between what the patient wants and what the therapist believes to be possible. Goals may change by mutual agreement during treatment but they should always be definite, practical and limited.

(7) All the stages above are a prelude to the work of treatment in which the patient changes his behaviour and gains some insight into his thinking and functioning. Change in behaviour usually precedes insight. Emphasis should be upon gradual change — achieving

little targets in sequence rather than attempting total coping instantaneously. As each goal is reached another attainable one is set.

(8) Reassurance is necessary. As the patient achieves minor goals, he is congratulated and it is pointed out to him how this contributes to the larger scheme of his learning to cope. The patient will require for himself genuine evidence of improvement.

(9) Attention must be paid to the relationship between patient and therapist. What are the needs for dependence of the patient upon the therapist and how can excessive dependence be avoided? The relevance of transference is recognised.

(10) When and how treatment should be terminated should be agreed at an early stage so that discharge is not felt as rejection by the patient. Before termination there should be an honest appraisal of the extent to which the goals have been achieved. Further goals should be agreed, to be achieved by the patient after treatment.

(11) Follow-up is the final stage of treatment. It is valuable therapeutically as it maintains the relationship of confidence of the patient in the therapist. It also serves as a monitor for goals set since termination. It is instructive for the therapist in evaluating his treatment methods and hence improving them.

In all patients with neuroses and personality disorders there is scope for improvement and there are usually treatment methods available which give hope for definite, although perhaps limited, improvement. It always involves active cooperation between patient and therapist. It has the twin goal of diminished symptoms and improved social relationships.

Bibliography

Anderson, S. and Hasler, J.C. (1979). Counselling in general practice. *J. R. Coll. gen. Practit.*, 29, 352-356

Balint, M. (1957). *The Doctor, his Patient and the Illness*, Pitman Medical, Tunbridge Wells

Balint, M. (1968). *The Basic Fault, Therapeutic Aspects of Regression*, Tavistock Publications, London

Bandura, A. (1978). Modelling. *Adv. Behav. Res. Ther.*, 1, 237-269

Beck, A., Rush, A., Shaw, B. and Emery, G. (1979). *Cognitive Therapy of Depression*, John Wiley, New York

Bloch, S. (1979). Assessment of patients for psychotherapy. *Br. J. Psychiat.*, 135, 193-208

Bowlby, J. (1969). *Attachment and Loss*, Hogarth Press, London

Committee on the Review of Medicines (1980). Systematic review of the benzodiazepines. *Br. med. J.*, 1, 910-912

Crowe, M.J. (1973). Conjoint marital therapy: advice or interpretation. *J. Psychosom. Res.*, 17, 309–15

Davies, M.H. (1976). The origins and practice of psychodrama. *Br. J. Psychiat.*, 129, 201–6

Dominian, J. (1968). *Marital Breakdown*, Penguin Books, Harmondsworth

Edwards, J.G. (1979). Overprescribing of psychotropic drugs. In: *Current Themes in Psychiatry*, 2 (Ed. Gaind, R.N. and Hudson, B.L.), MacMillan, London

Fairbairn, W.R.D. (1952). *Psychoanalytic Studies of the Personality: The Object Relation Theory of Personality*, Tavistock and Routledge & Kegan Paul, London

Fordham, F. (1953). *An Introduction to Jung's Psychology*, Penguin Books, Harmondsworth

Gelder, M. (1979). Behaviour therapy. In: *An Introduction to the Psychotherapies* (Bloch), Oxford University Press, London

Gillan, P. (1978). Treatment of sexual dysfunction. In: *Current Themes in Psychiatry*, 1 (Ed. Gaind, R.N. and Hudson, B.L.), MacMillan, London

Klein, M. (1948). *Contributions to Psycho-Analysis*, 1921–45, The Hogarth Press, London

Kogeorgos J. and Scott, D.F. (1981). Biofeedback and its clinical applications. *Br. J. Hosp. Med.*, 25, 601–605

Marks, I.M. (1979). Cure and care of neurosis. *Psychol. Med.*, 9, 629–660

Masters, W.H. and Johnson, V.E. (1970). *Human Sexual Inadequacy*, Churchill Livingstone, London

Menninger, K.A. (1958). *Theory of Psychoanalytic Technique*, Basic Books, New York

Rogers, C.R. (1967). *On becoming a Person. A Therapist's View of Psychotherapy*, Constable, London

Royal College of Psychiatrists (1979). *Alcohol & Alcholism*, Tavistock Publications, London

Sandler, J., Dare, C. and Holder, A. (1973). *The Patient and the Analyst: The Basis of the Psychoanalytic Process*, George Allen & Unwin, London

Sartre, J.P. (1943). *Being & Nothingness* (trans.), Methuen, London

Schultz, J.H., and Luthe, W. (1969). *Autogenic Therapy: 1 Autogenic Method*, Grune & Stratton, New York

Shepherd, M., Harwin, B.G., Depla, C. and Cairns, V. (1979). Social work and the primary care of mental disorder. *Psychol. Med.*, 9, 661–669

Snaith, R.P. (1981). *Clinical Neurosis*, Oxford University Press, Oxford

Sullivan, H.S. (1953). *The Interpersonal Theory of Psychiatry*, Tavistock Publications, London

Trethowan, W.H. (1975). Pills for personal problems. *Br. med. J.*, 4, 749–751

Tyrer, P. (1976). Towards rational therapy with monoamine oxidase inhibitors. *Br. J. Psychiat.*, 128, 354–360

Winnicott, W.D. (1958). *Collected Papers Through Paediatrics to Psychoanalysis*, Tavistock Publications, London

Yalom, I.D. (1975). *The Theory & Practice of Group Psychotherapy*, Basic Books, New York

Yalom, I.D. and Lieberman, M.A. (1971). A study of encounter group casualties. *Arch. gen. Psychiat.*, 25, 16–30

Further Reading (chapters 10 and 11)

Blackman, D. (1974). *Operant Conditioning: An Experimental Analysis of Behaviour*, Methuen, London

Bloch, S. (Ed.) (1979). *An Introduction to the Psychotherapies*, Oxford University Press, Oxford

Connolly, J. (1978). *Therapy Options in Psychiatry*, Pitman Medical, Tunbridge Wells

Crammer, J., Barraclough, B. and Heine, B. (1978). *The Use of Drugs in Psychiatry*, Gaskell, London

Frank, J.D. (1973). *Persuasion and Healing*, John Hopkins University Press

Gatchel, R.J. and Price, K.P. (1979). *Clinical Applications of Biofeedback: Appraisal and Status*, Pergamon Press, New York

Malan, D.H. (1979). *Individual Psychotherapy and the Science of Psychodynamics*, Butterworths, London

Minuchin, S. (1974). *Families and Family Therapy*, Tavistock Publications, London

Parry, R. (1975). *A Guide to Counselling and Basic Psychotherapy*, Churchill Livingstone, Edinburgh

Pincus, L. and Dare, C. (1978). *Secrets in the Family*, Faber & Faber, London

Silverstone, T. and Turner, P. (1978). *Drug Treatment in Psychiatry*, 2nd edn, Routledge & Kegan Paul, London

Storr, A. (1979). *The Art of Psychotherapy*, Secker & Warburg, London

Wolpe, J. (1973). *The Practice of Behaviour Therapy*, 2nd edn, Pergamon Press, New York

Index